I0838762

Eating For Health

Eating For Health

Discover the Scientifically Proven Foods that Combat and Reverse Disease

Victor Asher

Dedication

This book is dedicated to God for His grace and wisdom, to my family, to my beautiful readers who will find this book relevant to them, and to everyone who has loved, supported, and encouraged me along the way. I would not be in the position I am in today without your unshakable faith in me. I dedicate this book to all my readers' especially those who desire to stay healthy as this will sincerely be of importance to you all.

Table of Contents

Acknowledgement

I want to sincerely thank God for providing the means and insight that guided me during the writing of this book. I cannot forget my family members, whose encouragement and support have given me bravery and motivation throughout the process.

Thank you to my editor and publisher for their crucial advice and help in bringing this project to its successful conclusion. I would like to express my gratitude to everyone who so kindly contributed their time and knowledge to this project and added their wisdom. I want to express my gratitude to my friends as well, I appreciate all of your steadfast love and support throughout the journey.

I would like to express my gratitude to Walter C. Willett, M.D., G. Stephanie Rocket, supplementsglobal, medicaldaily, biocodex, taste.com.au, alchetron, seniorstoday.in, insularlife.com.ph and news-medical.net for their excellent images.

Finally, I extend my thanks to each and every one of you for purchasing and reading my work. I am thankful it met your needs and added to your knowledge. I sincerely value each and every one of you and think you're all fantastic.

Introduction

In today's fast-paced and often stressful world, maintaining good health and preventing disease have become top priorities for many individuals. The food we consume plays a critical role in our overall well-being, and scientific research has shown that certain foods possess remarkable properties that can combat and even reverse the onset of various diseases. By understanding the power of nutrition and making informed choices about what we eat, we can take control of our health and harness the potential of food as a powerful ally in disease prevention and management.

The concept of eating for health goes beyond mere sustenance; it is about nourishing our bodies with nutrient-dense foods that provide the essential components for optimal function and vitality. Scientific advancements have shed light on the profound impact that certain foods can have on our health, showing that they possess unique compounds and properties that actively combat disease at the cellular level. These foods have been found to possess anti-inflammatory, antioxidant, and immune-boosting properties, among other benefits, which contribute to their disease-fighting potential.

In this comprehensive guide, we will delve into the world of scientifically proven foods that combat and reverse disease. We will explore a wide range of health conditions, from chronic illnesses like heart disease, diabetes, and cancer to common ailments such as inflammation, cognitive decline, and digestive disorders. Each chapter will focus on specific diseases and the foods that have been scientifically studied and proven to be effective in preventing, managing, and even reversing these conditions.

Throughout this guide, we will uncover the science behind these disease-fighting foods, examining the bioactive compounds, vitamins, minerals, and other essential nutrients that contribute to their health benefits. We will explore the mechanisms by which these foods work, understanding how they combat inflammation, boost immune function, support healthy cellular processes, and promote overall well-being. Additionally, we will provide practical tips and strategies for incorporating these foods into your daily diet, ensuring that you can harness their disease-fighting potential and make positive changes to your health.

Eating for health is not about restrictive diets or quick fixes; it is a lifelong commitment to nourishing your body with the right foods to support optimal health and well-being. By embracing the scientifically proven foods that combat and reverse disease, you can take proactive steps towards a healthier future. Empower yourself with knowledge, make informed choices, and embark on a journey to transform your health through the power of nutrition. Get ready to discover the remarkable potential of food as medicine and embark on a path towards a vibrant and disease-free life.

Chapter 1

Overview on Nutrition

Nutrition is the process by which food is assimilated by living things so that they can develop, maintain themselves, and reproduce. It is also the process of ingesting, absorbing, and utilizing nutrients that the body needs for growth, development, and maintenance of life.

For the vast majority of living things, food has numerous purposes. For instance, it offers the substances that are digested to provide the energy necessary for the organism's various functions, such as the synthesis of cell components, movement and motility, excretion of waste products, and absorption and translocation of nutrients. Additionally, food offers the raw ingredients needed to create the live cell's structural and catalytic components.

The specific compounds that living things need as nourishment, how they produce these substances or get them from their environment, and the roles that these substances play within their cells are all different. However, there are commonalities that can be seen in the nutritional processes that occur throughout the living world as well as in the sorts of nutrients needed to support life.

People must eat a healthy diet that is rich in a range of nutrients, or the components of meals that nourish the body, in order to acquire adequate, proper nourishment. People who follow a healthy diet may do their regular physical and mental activities, maintain a healthy body weight, and reduce their risk of developing disease and disability. Body composition refers to the ratio of muscle to fat in the body.

According to the Dietary Guidelines for Americans 2020–2025 published by the United States Department of Agriculture (USDA), "A healthy dietary pattern consists of nutrient-dense forms of foods and beverages across all food groups, in recommended amounts, and within calorie limits." These recommendations state that the following are the essential components of a healthy eating pattern:

1. Vegetables of all colors, including red, orange, dark green, and starchy vegetables as well as beans, peas, and lentils.

2. Fruits, in particular whole fruit.

3. Grains, at least half of which are whole grain

4. Dairy products, such as lactose-free or fat-free milk, yogurt, and cheese, as well as fortified soy drinks and yogurt as substitutes.

5. Foods high in protein, such as lean meat, chicken, and eggs; Seafood, legumes like beans and lentils, and foods made of nuts, seeds, and soy.

6. Vegetable oils and oils found in foods like fish and nuts are among the oils.

One needs to follow nutritional requirements in order to avoid issues, due to the fact that obesity may occur when people eat too much. Toxic consequences (effects that hurt) may happen if people consume significant amounts of a few substances, typically vitamins or minerals. A nutritional deficiency disorder may come from undernutrition, which can happen when people don't get enough nutrients to stay healthy.

Types of Nutrition

When discussing nutrition, there are several types or categories that are commonly referred to. These categories help us understand the different components and aspects of a healthy and balanced diet.

Here are some of the key types of nutrition:

1. Macronutrients

Macronutrients are the major nutrients required by the body in large quantities to provide energy and support bodily functions. They include carbohydrates, proteins, and fats. Carbohydrates are the primary source of energy for the body, proteins are essential for growth, repair, and maintenance of body tissues, and fats play a role in energy storage, insulation, and the absorption of fat-soluble vitamins.

2. Micronutrients

Micronutrients are essential nutrients that the body needs in smaller quantities but are crucial for overall health. They include vitamins and minerals. Vitamins are organic compounds that are necessary for various biochemical processes in the body, such as energy production, immune function, and tissue repair. Minerals are inorganic substances that are essential for functions like bone health, nerve signaling, and enzyme activity.

3. Phytonutrients

Phytonutrients, also known as phytochemicals, are natural compounds found in plants. They are not considered essential nutrients but have been shown to have numerous health benefits. Phytonutrients have antioxidant, anti-inflammatory, and immune-boosting properties. Examples of phytonutrients include flavonoids, carotenoids, and polyphenols, which are found in colorful fruits and vegetables.

4. Functional Foods

Functional foods are foods that provide health benefits beyond basic nutrition. They are typically enriched with specific nutrients or bioactive compounds to promote health or prevent disease. Examples of functional foods include fortified cereals, probiotic yogurt, and omega-3 fatty acid-fortified eggs. These foods often have additional ingredients or modifications that target specific health concerns.

5. Whole Foods

Whole foods are minimally processed or unprocessed foods that are close to their natural state. They are rich in nutrients and typically have no added sugars, preservatives, or artificial additives. Whole foods (good source of dietary fibre) include fruits, vegetables, whole grains, lean meats, fish, legumes, and nuts. Consuming a diet rich in whole foods provides a wide range of nutrients and fiber.

6. Balanced Diet

A balanced diet refers to the consumption of a variety of foods from different food groups in appropriate proportions to meet the body's nutritional needs. It typically includes a combination of fruits, vegetables, whole grains, lean proteins, and healthy fats. A balanced diet ensures an adequate intake of essential nutrients and promotes overall health and well-being.

It's important to note that these types of nutrition are not mutually exclusive and often overlap. A healthy and balanced diet should encompass a combination of macronutrients, micronutrients, phytonutrients, and whole foods, while also considering individual dietary needs and goals. By understanding these different types of nutrition, individuals can make informed choices about their diet and optimize their nutritional intake for optimal health and well-being.

Water

While water is not typically classified as a type of nutrition, it plays a critical role in maintaining good health and is essential for our well-being. Water is a vital component of the human body, making up a significant portion of our cells, tissues, and organs. It is involved in various physiological processes and has several important functions.

1. Hydration

Water is crucial for maintaining proper hydration. It helps regulate body temperature, lubricates joints, and supports the transportation of nutrients and oxygen to cells. Staying properly hydrated is essential for optimal bodily functions and overall well-being.

2. Nutrient Absorption:

Water is necessary for the digestion and absorption of nutrients from the foods we eat. It helps break down food particles, aids in the absorption of nutrients in the digestive tract, and facilitates the movement of waste through the intestines.

3. Waste Removal

Water is essential for the excretion of waste products from the body. It helps flush out toxins and waste materials through urine, perspiration, and bowel movements. Sufficient water intake is crucial for maintaining healthy kidney function and preventing conditions such as kidney stones.

4. Body Fluid Balance

Water plays a vital role in maintaining the balance of body fluids. It helps regulate electrolyte levels, such as sodium and potassium, which are necessary for proper cell function, nerve impulses, and muscle contractions.

5. Energy Production

Water is involved in the metabolic processes that convert food into energy. It helps facilitate chemical reactions in the body, including those responsible for energy production and nutrient metabolism.

6. Brain Function

Proper hydration is important for optimal brain function. Research suggests that even mild dehydration can impair cognitive performance, attention, and mood. Drinking an adequate amount of water can help improve concentration, mental clarity, and overall brain function.

It is recommended to drink an adequate amount of water daily to maintain proper hydration. The exact amount can vary depending on factors such as age, activity level, climate, and overall health. While individual water needs may vary, a general guideline is to drink at least eight glasses (about 2 liters) of water per day. However, it's important to note that water needs can be met through various sources, including not just plain water but also other beverages and water-rich foods like fruits and vegetables.

In summary, while water is not classified as a type of nutrition, it is essential for maintaining good health and is involved in numerous vital functions in the body. Staying properly hydrated by drinking an adequate amount of water is crucial for optimal bodily functions, nutrient absorption, waste removal, and overall well-being.

When discussing the classes of food, it generally refers to the different categories of nutrients that are essential for the body's growth, development, and overall functioning. The main classes of food include carbohydrates, proteins, fats, vitamins, minerals, and water. Each class of food serves specific functions and provides unique benefits to the body. Let's explore each class of food in more detail:

1. Carbohydrates

Carbohydrates are the body's primary source of energy. They are found in foods such as grains, bread, pasta, rice, fruits, vegetables, and legumes. Carbohydrates are broken down into glucose, which is used by the body as a fuel for various activities, including physical exercise and brain function.

2. Proteins

Proteins are crucial for the growth, repair, and maintenance of body tissues. They are made up of amino acids and are found in foods like meat, fish, poultry, eggs, dairy products, legumes, and nuts. Proteins play a vital role in building and repairing muscles, producing enzymes and hormones, and supporting a healthy immune system.

3. Fats

Fats are an essential component of a healthy diet, providing energy, insulation, and cushioning for organs. They also assist in the absorption of fat-soluble vitamins. Healthy sources of fats include avocados, nuts, seeds, oily fish, and olive oil. It is important to choose healthier unsaturated fats while limiting saturated and trans fats.

4. Vitamins

Vitamins are organic compounds that are required in small amounts to support various bodily functions. They are essential for maintaining good health, immune function, and metabolism. Vitamins can be found in a wide range of foods, including fruits, vegetables, whole grains, dairy products, and meats. Examples of vitamins include vitamin C, vitamin A, vitamin D, and the B-complex vitamins.

5. Minerals

Minerals are inorganic substances that the body needs in small amounts for proper functioning. They are involved in numerous physiological processes, such as bone formation, nerve signaling, and enzyme activity. Common minerals include calcium, iron, potassium, zinc, and magnesium. Food sources of minerals include dairy products, leafy greens, legumes, meats, whole grains, and nuts.

6. Water

Water is not considered a nutrient, but it is essential for the body's survival. It plays a critical role in maintaining proper hydration, regulating body temperature, facilitating digestion and nutrient absorption, and eliminating waste products. Drinking an adequate amount of water and consuming water-rich foods like fruits and vegetables are essential for staying hydrated.

Understanding the different classes of food helps individuals make informed choices about their dietary intake. A balanced diet should include a variety of foods from each class, providing a diverse range of nutrients to support optimal health. It's important to note that individual dietary needs may vary based on factors such as age, sex, activity level, and specific health conditions. Consulting with a healthcare professional or registered dietitian can provide personalized guidance on meeting nutritional needs through appropriate food choices.

Food vs Nutrition

For us not to really get confused, I think we should understand the difference between food and nutrition, although they are closely related but distinct concepts.

Let's look at the difference between the two:

Food:

Food refers to any substance that is consumed by living organisms to provide energy, nourishment, and promote growth and development. It includes both solid and liquid substances that are ingested for sustenance. Food can be of plant or animal origin and is typically categorized into different groups, such as fruits, vegetables, grains, meats, dairy products, and more.

Food is consumed for various reasons, including satisfying hunger, enjoying flavors, cultural and social practices, and providing pleasure and satisfaction. Food encompasses a wide range of substances, including nutrients, as well as non-nutritive components like fiber, water, and bioactive compounds.

Nutrition:

Nutrition, on the other hand, is the scientific study of how food nourishes the body and affects health. It focuses on the nutrients and other substances present in food and how they are digested, absorbed, metabolized, and utilized by the body. Nutrition is concerned with the relationship between diet, health, and disease prevention.

It encompasses the study of macronutrients (carbohydrates, proteins, and fats), micronutrients (vitamins, minerals), phytonutrients, and other bioactive compounds found in food. Nutrition also involves understanding dietary patterns, nutritional requirements, and the impact of nutrition on growth, development, and overall well-being.

In summary, food refers to the substances we eat, while nutrition is the study of how those substances provide nourishment and impact our health. Food is the tangible, edible material, while nutrition is the science that investigates its composition, effects, and relationship with the body. By understanding nutrition, we can make informed choices about our food intake to promote optimal health and well-being.

Chapter 2

The Power of Nutrition in Combating and Reversing Disease

"The Power of Nutrition in Combating and Reversing Disease" talks about the significant impact that dietary choices can have on preventing, managing, and potentially reversing various diseases and health conditions. It emphasizes the potential of a well-balanced and nutrient-rich diet to support the body's natural healing processes and improve overall health outcomes.

This concept recognizes that the food we consume plays a fundamental role in our physiological functions and can either promote or hinder our well-being. A healthy diet, consisting of a variety of fruits, vegetables, whole grains, lean proteins, and healthy fats, provides essential nutrients that support the immune system, cellular repair, and the optimal functioning of our organs and systems.

Unhealthy eating habits, characterized by excessive consumption of processed foods, added sugars, unhealthy fats, and calorie-dense meals, have been strongly associated with the development and progression of these diseases. Conversely, adopting a nutritious diet can help prevent these conditions and improve management outcomes.

Furthermore, nutrition has the potential to reverse certain diseases under specific circumstances. For instance, lifestyle modifications that include dietary changes can lead to significant improvements in conditions like type 2 diabetes, where blood sugar control can be achieved through a well-managed diet. Similarly, adopting a diet that supports weight loss, reduces inflammation, and improves insulin sensitivity can positively impact conditions such as non-alcoholic fatty liver disease (NAFLD) and metabolic syndrome.

The power of nutrition in combating and reversing disease emphasizes the importance of making informed food choices and adopting healthy eating habits. However, it is essential to recognize that nutrition is not a standalone solution for all diseases, and individual needs may vary. Professional medical advice and guidance should be sought when managing specific conditions, and nutrition should be part of a comprehensive approach to health that includes physical activity, stress management, and other lifestyle factors.

Overall, by understanding and prioritizing the impact of diet on our well-being, individuals can take proactive steps towards better health and disease prevention.

Understanding the Impact of Food on Health

For current and future generations to remain healthy over the course of their lives, proper nutrition is crucial. A balanced diet lowers a child's chance of developing chronic diseases and supports healthy growth and development. Adults who consume a nutritious diet live longer and are less likely to develop obesity, heart disease, type 2 diabetes, or some malignancies. People with chronic diseases can control their conditions and prevent complications by maintaining a healthy diet.

When there aren't any healthy options, consumers could select items that are higher in calories and less nutritious. People from low-income areas and some racial and ethnic groups frequently do not have easy access to establishments that provide inexpensive, healthier foods.

The majority of Americans don't follow a healthy diet and consume excessive amounts of sodium, saturated fat, and sugar, which raises their risk of developing chronic diseases. For instance, less than 1 in 10 adults and adolescents consume adequate fruits and vegetables. Additionally, 5 out of 10 adults and 6 out of 10 children between the ages of 2 and 19 regularly consume sugary beverages.

Our diets can either give our bodies the energy they need to function correctly or they can have a negative impact on our health. The impact of what we eat on our mood, energy, and even risk of disease makes it crucial to be mindful of our dietary choices.

The impact of food on health is significant and plays a crucial role in overall well-being. The food we consume provides the nutrients our bodies need for energy, growth, and repair. However, not all foods are created equal, and our dietary choices can either promote good health or contribute to various health issues.

1. Nutritional Value

Food contains macronutrients (carbohydrates, proteins, and fats) and micronutrients (vitamins and minerals) essential for our body's proper functioning. A balanced diet that includes a variety of nutrient-dense foods ensures we receive adequate nutrition.

2. Energy and Weight Management

The calories we consume through food provide the energy required for daily activities. Eating a balanced diet can help maintain a healthy weight, preventing obesity-related conditions such as heart disease, type 2 diabetes, and certain cancers.

3. Disease Prevention

Certain foods, such as fruits, vegetables, whole grains, and lean proteins, are associated with a lower risk of chronic diseases. These foods are typically rich in vitamins, minerals, antioxidants, and fiber, which help protect against conditions like cardiovascular disease, stroke, and certain types of cancer.

4. Digestive Health

A diet high in fiber, obtained from fruits, vegetables, whole grains, and legumes, promotes healthy digestion and prevents conditions like constipation, diverticulosis, and hemorrhoids. Additionally, probiotic-rich foods (e.g., yogurt, sauerkraut) support a healthy gut microbiome, which plays a crucial role in overall health.

5. Mental Health

Emerging research suggests a link between diet and mental health. A diet rich in whole foods, omega-3 fatty acids (found in fatty fish, walnuts, and flaxseeds), and antioxidants (found in fruits and vegetables) may have a positive impact on mental well-being and reduce the risk of depression and anxiety.

6. Bone Health

Adequate calcium and vitamin D intake, obtained from dairy products, leafy greens, and sunlight exposure, is essential for maintaining strong bones and preventing conditions like osteoporosis.

7. Heart Health

A diet low in saturated and trans fats, cholesterol, and sodium, while high in fruits, vegetables, whole grains, lean proteins, and healthy fats (found in nuts, seeds, avocados, and olive oil), supports heart health and reduces the risk of cardiovascular diseases.

8. Food Allergies and Intolerances

Some individuals may have allergies or intolerances to certain foods, such as peanuts, shellfish, lactose, or gluten. Identifying and managing these conditions is crucial to avoid adverse health effects.

9. Hydration

Proper hydration is essential for various bodily functions. Drinking an adequate amount of water and consuming water-rich foods (e.g., fruits, vegetables, and soups) helps maintain optimal hydration levels.

10. Immune Function

Proper nutrition supports a healthy immune system, enabling the body to defend against infections and diseases. Key nutrients involved in immune function include vitamins A, C, E, zinc, and selenium.

11. Skin Health

Certain foods rich in antioxidants, vitamins, and healthy fats can contribute to healthier skin, reducing the risk of skin conditions and promoting a youthful appearance.

12. Blood Sugar Control

The selection of carbohydrates and the overall composition of meals can affect blood sugar levels. Balanced meals that include fiber-rich carbohydrates and lean proteins can help regulate blood sugar and prevent spikes.

13. Eye Health

Nutrients such as vitamin A, lutein, zeaxanthin, and omega-3 fatty acids play vital roles in maintaining good eye health and reducing the risk of age-related macular degeneration and cataracts.

It's important to note that individual nutritional needs may vary based on factors such as age, sex, activity level, and underlying health conditions. Consulting with a registered dietitian or healthcare professional can provide personalized guidance on dietary choices for optimal health.

The Science behind Disease Prevention and Reversal through Nutrition

"The Science behind Disease Prevention and Reversal through Nutrition" refers to the study and understanding of how specific dietary choices and nutritional interventions can help prevent and even reverse various diseases, or the understanding and application of scientific principles and evidence-based research that supports the use of nutrition as a means to prevent and reverse various diseases.

This concept recognizes that the food we consume plays a significant role in our overall health and well-being. It emphasizes the idea that adopting a healthy and balanced diet can have a profound impact on preventing the onset of diseases and even reversing certain conditions.

Disease prevention refers to strategies and practices aimed at reducing the risk of developing certain illnesses. It involves adopting healthy lifestyle habits, including a balanced and nutritious diet, regular exercise, and avoiding harmful behaviors like smoking or excessive alcohol consumption. By focusing on nutrition, one can make informed choices about the types and quantities of food they consume to minimize the likelihood of developing certain diseases.

Reversal through nutrition, pertains to the idea that proper nutrition can have a positive impact on existing diseases or conditions. In some cases, specific dietary modifications can potentially alleviate symptoms, slow down disease progression, or even reverse certain conditions altogether. This approach recognizes the influence of nutrition on overall health and its potential to support the body's natural healing processes.

The Science Behind" implies that there is scientific research and evidence supporting the relationship between nutrition and disease prevention or reversal. Researchers study various aspects of nutrition, such as the effects of specific nutrients, dietary patterns, or the role of certain food components (e.g., antioxidants, fiber, or phytochemicals) on disease processes. This scientific understanding forms the basis for recommendations and guidelines related to nutrition and health.

By studying the scientific literature, researchers and health professionals have gained insights into how specific nutrients and dietary patterns can influence the development and progression of diseases. They have identified associations between certain dietary factors and various health outcomes, including the prevention and management of conditions such as cardiovascular disease, diabetes, obesity, certain cancers, and others.

"The Science behind Disease Prevention and Reversal through Nutrition" encompasses a wide range of disciplines, including nutrition science, biochemistry, physiology, and epidemiology. It involves understanding how specific nutrients, bioactive compounds, and dietary patterns affect various biological processes and pathways within the body. This knowledge is then applied to develop evidence-based dietary guidelines and recommendations for disease prevention and management.

Numerous scientific studies have shown that a balanced and nutrient-rich diet can play a crucial role in preventing certain diseases. For example, a diet high in fruits, vegetables, whole grains, lean proteins, and healthy fats has been associated with a reduced risk of chronic conditions such as cardiovascular disease, type 2 diabetes, obesity, and certain types of cancer. On the other hand, a diet high in processed foods, added sugars, unhealthy fats, and excessive calories has been linked to an increased risk of these diseases. Similarly, dietary interventions have shown promise in managing conditions like hypertension, hyperlipidemia, and autoimmune disorders.

The mechanisms through which nutrition impacts disease prevention and reversal are diverse. Nutrients from food serve as building blocks for the body's cells, enzymes, and hormones, contributing to proper physiological functioning. Additionally, certain nutrients possess antioxidant and anti-inflammatory properties, which can protect against cellular damage and chronic inflammation, both of which are underlying factors in many diseases. Furthermore, a healthy diet can positively influence factors such as blood pressure, cholesterol levels, insulin sensitivity, and body weight, all of which are important for maintaining overall health and reducing the risk of disease.

It is important to note that while nutrition plays a significant role in disease prevention and reversal, it is not a standalone solution. Other factors such as physical activity, stress management, adequate sleep, and avoidance of harmful substances like tobacco and excessive alcohol also contribute to overall health and disease prevention.

In summary, the science behind disease prevention and reversal through nutrition encompasses a wide range of research exploring the relationship between dietary choices and health outcomes. By making informed decisions about food and adopting healthy eating habits, individuals can reduce their risk of developing various diseases and potentially improve their health outcomes if they already have a particular condition.

Chapter 3

Exploring Disease-Fighting Nutrients

Several nutrients have been associated with their potential to support the body's immune system and combat various diseases. Here are some examples:

1. Vitamin C

This antioxidant vitamin is known for its immune-boosting properties. It helps protect against oxidative stress, supports the production of white blood cells, and enhances immune cell function. Good sources of vitamin C include citrus fruits, strawberries, kiwi, bell peppers, and leafy greens.

2. Vitamin D

Adequate levels of vitamin D are crucial for a healthy immune system. It plays a role in modulating immune responses and reducing the risk of respiratory infections. Natural sources of vitamin D include sunlight exposure, fatty fish (e.g., salmon, mackerel), fortified dairy products, and egg yolks.

3. Zinc

Zinc is involved in immune cell development, function, and signaling. It helps regulate immune responses and supports wound healing. Food sources of zinc include oysters, red meat, poultry, beans, nuts, and whole grains.

4. Omega-3 fatty acids

These healthy fats have anti-inflammatory properties and play a role in immune regulation. They can help reduce the risk of chronic diseases such as cardiovascular disease and support overall immune function. Good sources of omega-3 fatty acids include fatty fish (e.g., salmon, sardines), flaxseeds, chia seeds, and walnuts.

5. Probiotics

These beneficial bacteria promote a healthy gut microbiome, which is essential for immune function. Probiotics can help strengthen the intestinal barrier, modulate immune responses, and reduce the risk of certain infections. Probiotic-rich foods include yogurt, kefir, sauerkraut, kimchi, and other fermented foods.

6. Antioxidants

Various antioxidants, such as vitamin E, selenium, and flavonoids, help combat oxidative stress and inflammation, thereby supporting immune health. Good sources of antioxidants include nuts, seeds, olive oil, green leafy vegetables, berries, and colorful fruits.

It's important to note that while these nutrients are associated with immune support and disease prevention, they should be consumed as part of a balanced and varied diet. Nutrients work synergistically, and overall dietary patterns are key to maintaining good health and supporting the body's defense against diseases.

Essential Vitamins and Minerals for Optimal Health

Maintaining optimal health requires a balanced intake of essential vitamins and minerals. While it's best to obtain these nutrients through a varied and balanced diet, sometimes supplementation may be necessary. Here are some key vitamins and minerals for optimal health:

1. Vitamin A

Essential for vision, immune function, and cell growth and differentiation. Sources include liver, fish oil, eggs, and orange and yellow fruits and vegetables.

2. Vitamin B complex

Includes several B vitamins like B1 (thiamine), B2 (riboflavin), B3 (niacin), B6 (pyridoxine), B9 (folate/folic acid), and B12 (cobalamin). They play crucial roles in energy production, brain function, metabolism, and red blood cell formation. Sources include whole grains, meat, fish, dairy products, legumes, and leafy greens.

3. Vitamin C

Acts as an antioxidant, supports the immune system, and aids in collagen synthesis. Good sources include citrus fruits, strawberries, kiwi, bell peppers, and leafy greens.

4. Vitamin D

Important for bone health, immune function, and calcium absorption. Our bodies can produce vitamin D when exposed to sunlight, but it can also be found in fatty fish, fortified dairy products, and egg yolks.

5. Vitamin E

An antioxidant that protects cells from damage and supports immune function. Good sources include nuts, seeds, vegetable oils, and leafy greens.

6. Vitamin K

Essential for blood clotting and bone health. Found in leafy greens, broccoli, Brussels sprouts, and some vegetable oils.

7. Calcium

Crucial for strong bones and teeth, muscle function, and nerve transmission. Dairy products, leafy greens, tofu, and fortified plant-based milk are good sources.

8. Iron

Required for the formation of red blood cells and oxygen transport. Found in red meat, poultry, fish, legumes, and fortified grains.

9. Magnesium

Important for over 300 enzymatic reactions in the body, including energy production, muscle function, and bone health. Good sources include nuts, seeds, whole grains, legumes, and leafy greens.

10. Zinc

Essential for immune function, wound healing, and DNA synthesis. Found in meat, shellfish, legumes, seeds, and nuts.

11. Potassium

Necessary for proper heart and muscle function, nerve transmission, and fluid balance. Bananas, citrus fruits, potatoes, leafy greens, and legumes are good sources.

12. Iodine

Essential for thyroid function and hormone production. Seafood, seaweed, iodized salt, and dairy products are sources of iodine.

Remember, it's always best to consult with a healthcare professional or a registered dietitian before starting any new supplements to determine your specific needs and potential interactions with medications or existing health conditions.

Antioxidants and Phytochemicals: Their Role in Combating Disease

Antioxidants and phytochemicals play a crucial role in combating disease by protecting our bodies against oxidative stress and inflammation. Here's a closer look at their functions and sources:

1. Antioxidants

Antioxidants are substances that help neutralize harmful free radicals, which are unstable molecules that can damage cells and contribute to various diseases, including cancer, heart disease, and neurodegenerative disorders. Antioxidants work by donating an electron to stabilize free radicals, thus preventing them from causing damage.

Common antioxidants include:

- Vitamin C

Found in citrus fruits, berries, bell peppers, and leafy greens.

- Vitamin E

Found in nuts, seeds, vegetable oils, and leafy greens.

- Beta-carotene

A precursor to vitamin A, found in orange and yellow fruits and vegetables, as well as leafy greens.

- Selenium

Found in Brazil nuts, fish, poultry, and whole grains.

2. Phytochemicals

Phytochemicals are natural compounds found in plant-based foods. They offer a wide range of health benefits, including antioxidant and anti-inflammatory properties. Phytochemicals have been associated with a reduced risk of chronic diseases such as cancer, cardiovascular disease, and age-related macular degeneration.

Common phytochemicals include:

- Flavonoids

Found in fruits, vegetables, tea, cocoa, and red wine.

- Carotenoids

Found in tomatoes, carrots, sweet potatoes, spinach, and kale.

- Resveratrol

Found in grapes, berries, and red wine.

- Isoflavones

Found in soybeans and soy products.

- Curcumin

Found in turmeric.

- Quercetin

Found in onions, apples, berries, and leafy greens.

These antioxidants and phytochemicals work together to combat disease through various mechanisms:

1. Neutralizing Free Radicals

Antioxidants donate electrons to free radicals, stabilizing them and preventing damage to cells and tissues.

2. Reducing Inflammation

Many phytochemicals have anti-inflammatory properties, which can help reduce chronic inflammation, a common underlying factor in many diseases.

3. Enhancing Immune Function

Antioxidants and phytochemicals support immune function, helping the body fight off infections and diseases.

4. Supporting DNA Repair

Some antioxidants aid in DNA repair, reducing the risk of genetic mutations and the development of certain diseases, including cancer.

It's important to note that while antioxidant-rich foods and phytochemicals are beneficial for health, the impact of isolated antioxidant supplements on disease prevention is still a topic of ongoing research. It's generally recommended to obtain these compounds through a varied and balanced diet rather than relying solely on supplements.

As always, consult with a healthcare professional or a registered dietitian for personalized advice on incorporating antioxidants and phytochemicals into your diet to support your specific health needs.

Omega-3 Fatty Acids: Promoting Heart Health and Reducing Inflammation

Omega-3 fatty acids are a type of polyunsaturated fat that play a crucial role in promoting heart health and reducing inflammation in the body. They are considered essential fats, meaning that our bodies cannot produce them and we must obtain them from our diet.

There are three main types of omega-3 fatty acids:

1. Eicosapentaenoic acid (EPA)

2. Docosahexaenoic acid (DHA)

3. Alpha-linolenic acid (ALA)

1. Eicosapentaenoic acid (EPA)

EPA is an omega-3 fatty acid that is primarily found in fatty fish, such as salmon, mackerel, and tuna. It is also synthesized from alpha-linolenic acid (ALA) in the body, although the conversion is limited. EPA is known for its role in reducing inflammation, promoting heart health, and supporting brain function. It has been studied for its potential benefits in reducing the risk of cardiovascular diseases and supporting mental well-being.

2. Docosahexaenoic acid (DHA)

DHA is another omega-3 fatty acid commonly found in fatty fish, as well as in fish oil supplements. It is a major structural component of the brain, eyes, and nervous system. DHA plays a crucial role in brain development and function, particularly during pregnancy and early childhood. It is also important for maintaining heart health, supporting cognitive function, and reducing inflammation. DHA is highly concentrated in the retina of the eye and is essential for optimal vision.

3. Alpha-linolenic acid (ALA)

ALA is an essential omega-3 fatty acid that is primarily obtained from plant sources such as flaxseeds, chia seeds, walnuts, and certain vegetable oils. Unlike EPA and DHA, ALA cannot be synthesized by the human body and must be obtained from the diet. Although ALA offers some health benefits, it is important to note that the conversion of ALA to EPA and DHA in the body is limited. Therefore, consuming direct sources of EPA and DHA from fish or algal oil is often recommended for optimal omega-3 intake.

Each of these omega-3 fatty acids plays a vital role in supporting various aspects of health, including heart health, brain function, and reducing inflammation. It's important to include a variety of omega-3-rich foods in your diet or consider supplementation, based on your specific dietary needs and health goals.

Here's how omega-3 fatty acids benefit heart health and help reduce inflammation:

1. Heart Health

Omega-3 fatty acids have been shown to have several beneficial effects on heart health, including:

- Lowering triglyceride levels: Omega-3s can help reduce levels of triglycerides, a type of fat in the blood that, when elevated, increases the risk of heart disease.

- Reducing blood pressure: Studies have suggested that omega-3 fatty acids may help lower blood pressure levels, thereby reducing the risk of hypertension and related cardiovascular conditions.

- Preventing plaque buildup: Omega-3s can help prevent the formation of plaque in arteries, reducing the risk of atherosclerosis and heart disease.

- Modulating heart rhythm: Omega-3 fatty acids have been shown to have antiarrhythmic effects, helping to stabilize the heart's electrical activity and reducing the risk of abnormal heart rhythms.

2. Inflammation Reduction

Omega-3 fatty acids possess anti-inflammatory properties that can help reduce chronic inflammation in the body. Chronic inflammation is associated with a wide range of diseases, including heart disease, rheumatoid arthritis, and inflammatory bowel disease. By reducing inflammation, omega-3s may help alleviate symptoms and improve overall health.

Good dietary sources of omega-3 fatty acids include:

- Fatty fish: Cold-water fatty fish such as salmon, mackerel, sardines, trout, and tuna are rich in EPA and DHA.

- Algal oil: A vegetarian source of omega-3s derived from algae, which is a source of EPA and DHA.

- Flaxseeds and chia seeds: These seeds are high in ALA, a plant-based omega-3 fatty acid. However, the conversion of ALA to EPA and DHA in the body is limited.

- Walnuts: They are a good plant-based source of ALA.

- Omega-3 fortified foods: Some food products, such as eggs, milk, and yogurt, may be fortified with omega-3 fatty acids.

For individuals who don't consume enough omega-3-rich foods, supplementation with fish oil or algal oil capsules can be an option. However, it's important to consult with a healthcare professional before starting any new supplements to determine the appropriate dosage and ensure they fit into your overall health plan.

In all, omega-3 fatty acids are essential for heart health and have anti-inflammatory effects in the body. Including a variety of omega-3-rich foods in your diet can contribute to overall well-being and reduce the risk of chronic diseases.

Chapter 4

The Mediterranean Diet: A Blueprint for Health

The Mediterranean diet is a dietary pattern inspired by the traditional eating habits of countries bordering the Mediterranean Sea, such as Greece, Italy, Spain, and Morocco. The traditional foods and eating styles of Portugal, southern Spain, southern Italy, Crete, and much of the rest of Greece that were first made known to the world in the early 1960s are the inspiration for the Mediterranean diet. This sets it apart from Mediterranean food, which is native to and develops naturally in Mediterranean nations.

The "Mediterranean diet" was later proved and improved based on the findings of several scientific investigations, despite being inspired by a particular time and place. It has gained recognition as a blueprint for health due to its association with numerous health benefits and lower risk of chronic diseases.

The main components of this diet include a proportionately high intake of unprocessed grains, legumes, olive oil, fruits, and vegetables, as well as a moderate intake of fish, dairy products (primarily cheese and yogurt), and meat products. Olive oil has been investigated as a potential health factor for lowering mortality from all causes and the chance of developing chronic diseases.

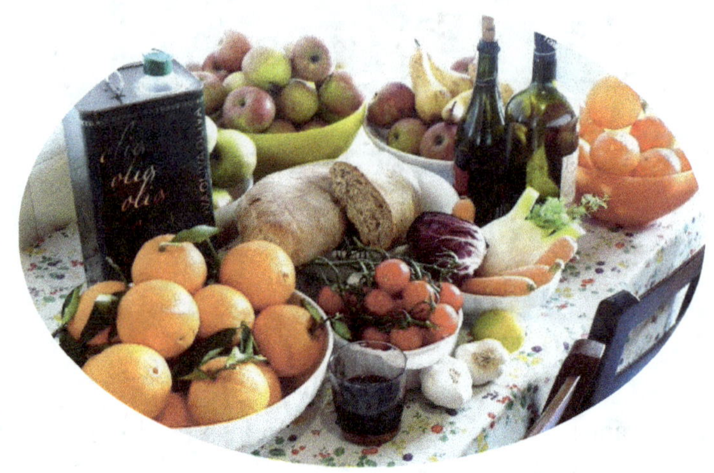

In observational studies, the Mediterranean diet is linked to a decline in overall mortality. Evidence indicating the Mediterranean diet reduces the risk of heart disease and early death was reported in 2017 in the European Journal of Clinical Nutrition. The Mediterranean diet may aid obese people in losing weight. The DASH diet, vegetarianism, and the Mediterranean diet are the three healthy diets advocated in the 2015-2020 Dietary Guidelines for Americans. Two of the primary sources for the MIND diet recommendations are the Mediterranean and DASH diets.

It is good to note that the Mediterranean diet is not the same as the cultural practices that UNESCO listed in 2010 under the heading "Mediterranean diet" on the Representative List of the Intangible Cultural Heritage of Humanity: "a set of skills, knowledge, rituals, symbols, and traditions concerning crops, harvesting, fishing, animal husbandry, conservation, processing, cooking, and especially the sharing and consumption."

Here are some key characteristics and benefits of the Mediterranean diet:

1. Plant-based focus

The Mediterranean diet emphasizes a high consumption of fruits, vegetables, whole grains, legumes, nuts, and seeds. These foods provide a rich array of vitamins, minerals, fiber, and antioxidants, which contribute to overall health and well-being.

2. Healthy fats

Instead of saturated and trans fats, the Mediterranean diet favors healthier fats, such as olive oil, avocados, and nuts. These sources of monounsaturated and polyunsaturated fats, including omega-3 fatty acids, have been linked to a reduced risk of heart disease and improved cholesterol levels.

3. Fish and lean protein

Fish, particularly fatty fish like salmon, mackerel, and sardines, are key components of the Mediterranean diet due to their omega-3 fatty acid content. It promotes heart health and supports brain function. Poultry, eggs, and dairy products, including yogurt and cheese, are consumed in moderation, while red meat is limited.

4. Moderate consumption of red wine

In moderation, red wine is often consumed with meals in the Mediterranean diet, primarily in countries like Greece and Italy. It is believed that the moderate consumption of red wine, which contains antioxidants like resveratrol, may contribute to heart health. However, it's important to note that excessive alcohol consumption is harmful and should be avoided.

5. Herbs and spices

The Mediterranean diet relies on herbs and spices to add flavor to meals, reducing the need for excessive salt and unhealthy condiments. Common herbs and spices used include basil, oregano, rosemary, garlic, and lemon.

The Mediterranean diet has been associated with numerous health benefits, including:

- **Reduced risk of heart disease:** The emphasis on healthy fats, whole grains, fruits, vegetables, and fish contributes to lower rates of cardiovascular diseases.

- **Improved weight management:** The high fiber content, nutrient-dense foods, and focus on portion control can support healthy weight management.

- **Lower risk of type 2 diabetes**: The Mediterranean diet is associated with improved insulin sensitivity and lower rates of type 2 diabetes.

- **Cognitive health**: The diet's emphasis on fruits, vegetables, whole grains, healthy fats, and fish has been linked to a reduced risk of cognitive decline and neurodegenerative diseases like Alzheimer's.

- **Reduced inflammation:** The abundant antioxidants, omega-3 fatty acids, and plant-based foods in the diet contribute to its anti-inflammatory effects.

It's important to note that the Mediterranean diet is not just about the individual components but also the overall dietary pattern and lifestyle, including regular physical activity, social engagement, and mindful eating. As with any diet, it's best to personalize it based on individual needs and preferences, and consult with a healthcare professional or a registered dietitian for guidance.

The Mediterranean diet food pyramid, summarizing the pattern of eating associated with this diet.

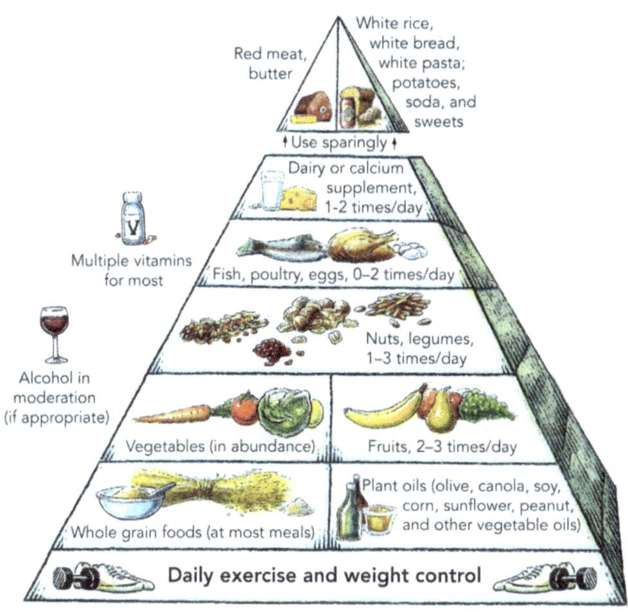

Unveiling the Science behind the Mediterranean Diet

The Mediterranean diet is a dietary pattern that originated in the Mediterranean region and is known for its health benefits. It has been extensively studied and has shown positive effects on various aspects of health, including heart health, weight management, and longevity.

The science behind the Mediterranean diet involves several key components:

1. High consumption of fruits, vegetables, and whole grains

These foods are rich in essential vitamins, minerals, and fiber. They provide antioxidants and phytochemicals, which have been associated with reduced risk of chronic diseases, such as heart disease and certain types of cancer.

2. Emphasis on healthy fats

The Mediterranean diet includes moderate amounts of healthy fats, primarily from olive oil, nuts, and seeds. These fats are high in monounsaturated and polyunsaturated fats, including omega-3 fatty acids. These fats have been shown to have anti-inflammatory properties and can help improve cholesterol levels and reduce the risk of heart disease.

3. Moderate consumption of dairy products, poultry, and eggs

The Mediterranean diet includes moderate amounts of these protein sources. It promotes choosing low-fat options and limiting intake of red meat, which is high in saturated fats and associated with an increased risk of heart disease.

4. Regular consumption of fish and seafood

The Mediterranean diet encourages the consumption of fish, particularly fatty fish like salmon, sardines, and mackerel. These fish are rich in omega-3 fatty acids, which have been shown to have numerous health benefits, including reducing inflammation and improving heart health.

5. Limited intake of processed foods and added sugars

The Mediterranean diet focuses on whole, unprocessed foods and discourages the consumption of processed foods, refined grains, and added sugars. This helps reduce the intake of unhealthy fats, excessive sodium, and empty calories.

6. Moderate consumption of alcohol, primarily in the form of red wine

The Mediterranean diet allows for moderate alcohol consumption, primarily in the form of red wine during meals. However, it's important to note that excessive alcohol consumption can have negative health effects, and moderation is key.

The science behind the Mediterranean diet suggests that its beneficial effects on health can be attributed to the combination of these dietary components. It promotes a nutrient-rich, balanced eating pattern that is associated with reduced inflammation, improved blood lipid profiles, better blood sugar control, and overall cardiovascular health. Additionally, the diet is often accompanied by a healthy lifestyle, including regular physical activity and social engagement, which further contributes to its positive effects.

Key Components of the Mediterranean Diet

The key components of the Mediterranean diet are as follows:

1. Abundant intake of fruits and vegetables

The Mediterranean diet emphasizes consuming a wide variety of fruits and vegetables, which are excellent sources of vitamins, minerals, fiber, and antioxidants.

2. Whole grains

Whole grains like whole wheat, brown rice, oats, and quinoa are staples of the Mediterranean diet. These provide complex carbohydrates, fiber, and essential nutrients.

3. Healthy fats

The diet incorporates healthy fats, primarily in the form of olive oil. Olive oil is rich in monounsaturated fats, which are beneficial for heart health. Other sources of healthy fats in the Mediterranean diet include nuts, seeds, and avocados.

4. Legumes

Legumes such as beans, lentils, chickpeas, and peas are an important part of the Mediterranean diet. They are excellent sources of plant-based protein, fiber, and various minerals.

5. Fish and seafood

The Mediterranean diet encourages the consumption of fish and seafood, particularly fatty fish like salmon, sardines, and mackerel. These are rich in omega-3 fatty acids, which have numerous health benefits.

6. Moderate consumption of poultry, eggs, and dairy

The Mediterranean diet includes moderate amounts of poultry, eggs, and dairy products like yogurt and cheese. These provide protein, calcium, and other essential nutrients.

7. Limited intake of red meat

Red meat is consumed sparingly in the Mediterranean diet. When consumed, it is usually in smaller portions and as an accompaniment rather than the main focus of a meal.

8. Herbs and spices for flavoring

The Mediterranean diet relies on herbs and spices, such as garlic, basil, rosemary, and oregano, for flavoring rather than excessive salt or high-sodium seasonings.

9. Moderate consumption of red wine

In moderation, red wine is often enjoyed with meals in the Mediterranean diet. However, it's important to note that excessive alcohol consumption can have negative health effects, and moderation is key.

10. Regular physical activity and social connections

While not strictly a dietary component, the Mediterranean diet is often accompanied by an active lifestyle and a focus on socializing with family and friends. These factors contribute to overall well-being.

It's important to note that the Mediterranean diet is a flexible and adaptable eating pattern, and the specific foods and proportions may vary depending on regional and cultural differences.

Research on the Diet's Impact on Disease Prevention and Reversal

Research on the impact of diet on disease prevention and reversal is a dynamic and evolving field. Numerous studies have investigated the relationship between diet and various diseases, and while there is still much to learn, there is a growing body of evidence suggesting that diet plays a crucial role in both the prevention and reversal of certain diseases.

Here are some key areas of research:

1. Cardiovascular Disease

Multiple studies have shown that a healthy diet, such as the Mediterranean diet or the Dietary Approaches to Stop Hypertension (DASH) diet, can reduce the risk of developing cardiovascular diseases like heart disease and stroke. These diets emphasize fruits, vegetables, whole grains, lean proteins (such as fish and poultry), and healthy fats (such as olive oil). They also limit the intake of red meat, processed foods, and sugary beverages.

2. Type 2 Diabetes

Diet has a significant impact on the development and management of type 2 diabetes. Research has demonstrated that a healthy diet, focusing on whole grains, legumes, fruits, vegetables, lean proteins, and healthy fats, can help prevent the onset of type 2 diabetes. In individuals with the condition, a well-balanced diet combined with weight management can improve blood sugar control and potentially lead to disease reversal.

3. Obesity

Obesity is a risk factor for numerous diseases, including cardiovascular disease, type 2 diabetes, certain cancers, and more. Dietary interventions, such as calorie restriction, balanced macronutrient distribution, and increased physical activity, are commonly recommended for weight loss and obesity management. Sustainable weight loss achieved through a healthy diet can significantly reduce the risk of obesity-related diseases.

4. Cancer

While the relationship between diet and cancer is complex, research suggests that certain dietary patterns can influence cancer risk. A diet rich in fruits, vegetables, whole grains, and lean proteins, while low in processed meats, sugary foods, and refined grains, appears to have a protective effect against various cancers. However, it's important to note that individual dietary factors may have different effects on specific types of cancer.

5. Neurodegenerative Diseases

Emerging evidence suggests that specific diets, such as the Mediterranean diet and the MIND diet (a combination of the Mediterranean and DASH diets), may help reduce the risk of neurodegenerative diseases like Alzheimer's disease. These diets emphasize plant-based foods, healthy fats, lean proteins, and limited intake of red meat, processed foods, and added sugars.

6. Inflammatory Diseases

Chronic inflammation is linked to several diseases, including rheumatoid arthritis, inflammatory bowel disease, and autoimmune disorders. Research suggests that certain diets, such as the anti-inflammatory diet or Mediterranean-style diets, which include plenty of fruits, vegetables, whole grains, healthy fats (such as olive oil), and fish, while limiting processed foods, refined sugars, and saturated fats, may help reduce inflammation and improve symptoms in these conditions.

7. Gastrointestinal Health

Diet plays a crucial role in maintaining a healthy gut microbiome, which is essential for digestive health. Emerging research suggests that a diet rich in fiber from whole grains, fruits, and vegetables, along with fermented foods (such as yogurt and sauerkraut) and prebiotics (such as onions and garlic), can promote a diverse and beneficial gut microbiota. This may help prevent gastrointestinal conditions, such as irritable bowel syndrome (IBS) and inflammatory bowel disease (IBD).

8. Bone Health

Adequate nutrient intake, particularly calcium and vitamin D, is essential for maintaining bone health and preventing conditions like osteoporosis. A diet that includes calcium-rich foods like dairy products, leafy greens, and fortified products, along with sufficient vitamin D from sources like fatty fish and sunlight exposure, can support optimal bone health and reduce the risk of fractures.

9. Mental Health

There is growing evidence suggesting a link between diet and mental health. Certain dietary patterns, such as the Mediterranean diet and the DASH diet, rich in fruits, vegetables, whole grains, lean proteins, and healthy fats, have been associated with a lower risk of depression and cognitive decline. On the other hand, diets high in processed and sugary foods have been linked to an increased risk of mental health disorders.

It's important to note that while diet plays a crucial role in disease prevention and reversal, it should be considered as part of a comprehensive approach to health that includes other lifestyle factors, such as regular physical activity, stress management, adequate sleep, and avoiding smoking and excessive alcohol consumption.

Additionally, individual responses to diet can vary, and personalized approaches may be necessary for optimal health outcomes. Consultation with healthcare professionals or registered dietitians is recommended for personalized dietary recommendations.

Chapter 5

Superfoods: Nature's Disease Fighters

Superfoods are nutrient-dense foods celebrated for their exceptional health benefits and disease-fighting properties. Packed with a wide range of vitamins, minerals, antioxidants, and other beneficial compounds, they offer a natural way to boost overall well-being and help prevent various illnesses. From antioxidant-rich berries to vitamin-packed leafy greens, superfoods have been associated with a reduced risk of chronic diseases such as heart disease, cancer, diabetes, and neurodegenerative disorders. By incorporating superfoods into your diet, you can tap into the power of nature to optimize nutrition and improve your health.

While superfoods are not magical cure-alls, they can play a significant role in a well-balanced diet and a healthy lifestyle. They can strengthen the immune system, support cardiovascular health, aid in digestion, reduce inflammation, and contribute to weight management. However, it's important to remember that no single food can replace a varied and nutritious diet as a whole. The key is to incorporate a diverse range of fruits, vegetables, whole grains, lean proteins, and other healthy foods to provide comprehensive nourishment. By embracing superfoods as part of a holistic approach to eating, you can proactively support your body's natural defense systems and promote optimal health.

Note, superfoods and their potential benefits should be considered in the context of an overall healthy lifestyle, including regular physical activity and a balanced diet. It is always advisable to consult with a healthcare professional or a registered dietitian for personalized guidance on incorporating superfoods into your diet based on your individual health needs and goals.

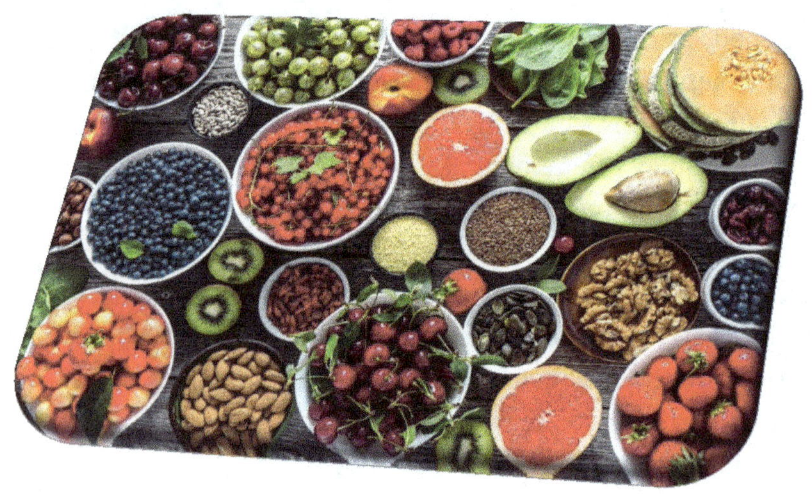

Introduction to Superfoods and Their Nutritional Benefits

While the term "superfoods" is not a scientific classification, it is commonly used to refer to nutrient-dense foods that are considered to have exceptional health benefits due to their high concentration of vitamins, minerals, antioxidants, and other beneficial compounds, or foods that provide a significant boost to overall health and well-being.

Superfoods come from a variety of plant and animal sources, and each superfood has its unique nutritional profile and health benefits. Here are some popular examples of superfoods and their nutritional benefits:

1. Blueberries

Blueberries are packed with antioxidants, specifically anthocyanins, which help protect the body against damage from free radicals. They are also a good source of fiber, vitamin C, vitamin K, and manganese, supporting heart health, brain function, and reducing inflammation.

2. Kale

Kale is a leafy green vegetable that is rich in vitamins A, C, and K, as well as minerals like calcium and potassium. It is also a great source of antioxidants and fiber, promoting healthy digestion, reducing cholesterol levels, and supporting bone health.

3. Salmon

Salmon is a fatty fish that is an excellent source of omega-3 fatty acids, which are beneficial for heart health and reducing inflammation. It also provides high-quality protein, vitamin D, and several essential minerals.

4. Quinoa

Quinoa is a grain-like seed that is gluten-free and rich in protein, fiber, and various minerals such as magnesium, iron, and zinc. It is considered a complete protein as it contains all nine essential amino acids, making it an excellent choice for vegetarians and vegans.

5. Chia seeds

Chia seeds are tiny black seeds that are a powerhouse of nutrients. They are an excellent source of fiber, omega-3 fatty acids, antioxidants, and minerals like calcium and magnesium. Chia seeds can help regulate blood sugar levels, support digestion, and promote satiety.

6. Greek yogurt

Greek yogurt is a creamy and protein-rich dairy product. It is lower in lactose and contains probiotics, which are beneficial for gut health. Greek yogurt also provides calcium, vitamin B12, and other essential nutrients.

7. Spinach

Spinach is a leafy green vegetable that is loaded with vitamins A, C, and K, as well as folate, iron, and antioxidants. It supports eye health, strengthens the immune system, and helps maintain healthy blood pressure levels.

8. Turmeric

Turmeric is a spice known for its vibrant yellow color and active compound called curcumin. Curcumin has powerful anti-inflammatory and antioxidant properties, making turmeric beneficial for reducing inflammation, boosting brain health, and supporting joint function.

9. Mushrooms

Mushrooms, such as shiitake, maitake, and reishi, are rich in antioxidants, vitamins, minerals, and bioactive compounds. They have shown immune-enhancing properties, potential anti-cancer effects, and the ability to modulate inflammation and support cardiovascular health.

10. Spirulina

Spirulina is a blue-green algae that is highly nutritious, containing protein, vitamins, minerals, and antioxidants. It has been studied for its potential immune-boosting, anti-inflammatory, and cholesterol-lowering effects. Spirulina may also have protective effects against oxidative stress-related diseases.

11. Avocados

Avocados are a good source of healthy fats, fiber, vitamins (such as vitamin K, vitamin C, and vitamin E), and minerals. They have been associated with various health benefits, including improved cardiovascular health, weight management, and enhanced absorption of nutrients from other foods.

12. Walnuts

Walnuts are a nutrient-dense nut rich in omega-3 fatty acids, antioxidants, and fiber. They have been associated with improved heart health, cognitive function, and reduced inflammation. Consuming walnuts has also been linked to a lower risk of certain cancers, such as breast and colorectal cancer.

13. Ginger

Ginger is a root spice known for its anti-inflammatory and digestive properties. It contains bioactive compounds, such as gingerol, which have demonstrated antioxidant, anti-cancer, and anti-inflammatory effects. Ginger may also help alleviate nausea and support gastrointestinal health.

14. Garlic

Garlic is known for its potent antimicrobial, anti-inflammatory, and cardiovascular benefits. It contains sulfur compounds that have shown potential in reducing blood pressure, improving cholesterol levels, and boosting immune function.

15. Green tea

Green tea is rich in catechins, which are powerful antioxidants that have been associated with a reduced risk of cardiovascular disease, certain cancers, and improved brain health. Green tea also contains caffeine and L-theanine, which can enhance cognitive function and promote relaxation.

16. Dark chocolate

Dark chocolate with a high cocoa content is rich in flavonoids, which have antioxidant and anti-inflammatory properties. Consuming dark chocolate in moderation has been associated with improved heart health, blood pressure regulation, and cognitive function.

17. Pomegranate

Pomegranates are packed with antioxidants, particularly punicalagins, which have shown anti-inflammatory and anti-cancer effects. Consuming pomegranate or its juice has been associated with improved heart health, reduced oxidative stress, and potential benefits against certain types of cancer.

18. Tomatoes

Tomatoes are rich in lycopene, a powerful antioxidant that gives them their red color. Lycopene has been studied for its potential in reducing the risk of certain cancers, particularly prostate cancer. Tomatoes also provide vitamin C, potassium, and other beneficial compounds.

It's important to note that while superfoods can be a part of a healthy diet, they should not replace a balanced and varied eating plan. Incorporating a wide range of nutrient-rich foods into your diet, including superfoods, can help optimize your overall nutritional intake and promote better health and well-being.

Incorporating superfoods into your daily diet can be a great way to enhance your overall nutritional intake and promote better health.

Here are some tips on how to include superfoods in your daily meals:

1. Plan your meals

Take some time to plan your meals in advance, incorporating a variety of superfoods. This will help ensure that you have a balanced and nutrient-rich diet throughout the week.

2. Start your day with a superfood breakfast

Include superfoods like berries, chia seeds, or Greek yogurt in your breakfast. You can add berries to your oatmeal or yogurt, sprinkle chia seeds on your cereal, or incorporate nutrient-dense greens like spinach into your omelets or smoothies.

3. Snack on superfoods

Instead of reaching for unhealthy snacks, opt for superfood snacks. You can have a handful of nuts like walnuts or almonds, munch on carrot sticks with hummus, or enjoy a piece of dark chocolate with a high cocoa content.

4. Load up on vegetables

Include a variety of vegetables in your meals. Leafy greens like kale and spinach, cruciferous vegetables like broccoli and cauliflower, and colorful vegetables like bell peppers and tomatoes are all excellent choices.

5. Incorporate whole grains and seeds

Replace refined grains with whole grains like quinoa, brown rice, or whole wheat bread. These provide more fiber, vitamins, and minerals. Additionally, add seeds like flaxseeds or pumpkin seeds to your salads, smoothies, or yogurt for added nutritional benefits.

6. Experiment with herbs and spices

Use herbs and spices like turmeric, ginger, garlic, and cinnamon to enhance the flavor and nutritional value of your dishes. These ingredients are not only delicious but also have potential health benefits.

7. Make superfood salads

Create nutrient-packed salads by combining a variety of superfoods. Include ingredients like leafy greens, colorful vegetables, berries, avocado, nuts, and seeds. Drizzle with a healthy dressing made from olive oil and lemon juice or vinegar.

8. Cook with superfood ingredients

Incorporate superfoods into your cooking. For example, add mushrooms to stir-fries or soups, use spirulina powder in smoothies or homemade energy bars, or include avocado in sandwiches or as a topping for toast.

9. Stay hydrated with superfood-infused beverages

Prepare superfood-infused beverages like green tea, matcha lattes, or herbal teas with ingredients like ginger, turmeric, or lemon for added health benefits.

Remember, it's important to include a variety of superfoods in your diet and not rely solely on a few specific ones. By diversifying your food choices, you can ensure you're getting a wide range of nutrients and maximizing the potential health benefits.

Chapter 6

The Plant-Based Revolution: Harnessing the Power of Plants for Health

The plant-based revolution is a growing movement that emphasizes the importance of incorporating more plant foods into our diets for improved health and well-being. This approach focuses on harnessing the power of plants to provide essential nutrients, promote disease prevention, and support overall vitality.

A plant-based diet emphasizes whole grains, fruits, vegetables, legumes, nuts, and seeds while minimizing or eliminating animal products. By prioritizing plant foods, individuals can benefit from the abundance of vitamins, minerals, antioxidants, and fiber they provide. Research suggests that a plant-based diet can help reduce the risk of chronic diseases such as heart disease, diabetes, obesity, and certain types of cancer.

Embracing a plant-based lifestyle not only supports personal health but also has positive implications for environmental sustainability and animal welfare. By choosing plant-based options, individuals contribute to reducing their ecological footprint and promoting a more compassionate approach to food choices.

The plant-based revolution is about more than just dietary changes; it represents a shift towards a more mindful and conscious way of living. It encourages individuals to explore creative and delicious plant-based recipes, discover new flavors and textures, and develop a deeper connection with nature and the food we consume.

As with any dietary change, it's important to approach the plant-based revolution with informed choices and balance. Consulting with a healthcare professional or a registered dietitian can provide personalized guidance to ensure nutritional needs are met and to address any individual concerns.

By embracing the plant-based revolution, individuals can harness the power of plants to nourish their bodies, support their health goals, and contribute to a more sustainable and compassionate world.

Plant-Based Diets and Their Impact on Disease Prevention

Plant-based diets are dietary patterns that prioritize the consumption of plant foods while minimizing or excluding animal products. These diets revolve around whole grains, fruits, vegetables, legumes, nuts, and seeds as the primary sources of nutrition.

Plant-based diets are characterized by a focus on plant foods as the central component of meals, while reducing or eliminating the consumption of animal products. These diets have gained popularity due to their potential health benefits, environmental sustainability, and ethical considerations.

In a plant-based diet, the primary sources of nutrition come from whole grains, fruits, vegetables, legumes, nuts, and seeds. These foods provide essential nutrients such as vitamins, minerals, fiber, and phytochemicals. Plant-based diets tend to be higher in fiber and lower in saturated fat and cholesterol compared to diets that include more animal products.

The specific type of plant-based diet can vary based on individual preferences and beliefs. Vegan diets exclude all animal products, while vegetarian diets eliminate meat and poultry but may include dairy and/or eggs. Flexitarian or semi-vegetarian diets allow for occasional consumption of meat, poultry, or fish, while pescatarian diets include fish and seafood but exclude other types of meat.

Plant-based diets have been associated with numerous health benefits, including a reduced risk of chronic diseases such as heart disease, type 2 diabetes, certain cancers, and obesity. They also tend to be more environmentally sustainable, as plant foods generally require fewer resources and produce fewer greenhouse gas emissions compared to animal-based foods.

When following a plant-based diet, it is important to ensure proper nutrient intake, particularly for nutrients that may be more limited in plant-based sources, such as vitamin B12, iron, calcium, and omega-3 fatty acids. Consulting with a healthcare professional or a registered dietitian can provide personalized guidance to ensure nutritional needs are met while following a plant-based diet.

There are different types of plant-based diets, including:

1. Vegan Diet

A vegan diet excludes all animal products, including meat, poultry, fish, dairy, eggs, and honey. It focuses solely on plant foods and may incorporate alternatives like plant-based milk, tofu, tempeh, and seitan.

Vegans can include plant-based sources of protein such as tofu, tempeh, seitan, and lentils to satisfy their protein demands. In place of dairy milk, you can use plant-based milk substitutes like soy, almond, and oat milk. There are other vegan alternatives that can mimic the tastes and textures of conventional animal-based goods, such nutritional yeast, plant-based cheeses, and egg substitutes.

All the nutrients required for a healthy and balanced lifestyle can be obtained through a well-planned vegan diet. However, some minerals, like vitamin B12, iron, calcium, and omega-3 fatty acids, that are frequently present in animal products should be taken into consideration by vegans. To ensure correct nutrient balance, they may need to guarantee enough consumption through fortified meals or supplements and seek advice from a healthcare provider or certified dietitian.

2. Vegetarian Diet

Vegetarian diets eliminate meat and poultry but may include animal-derived products such as dairy and eggs. There are variations within the vegetarian diet, including lacto-vegetarian (includes dairy), ovo-vegetarian (includes eggs), and lacto-ovo-vegetarian (includes both dairy and eggs).

Here are the common variations of a vegetarian diet:

- Lacto-Vegetarian: Lacto-vegetarians include dairy products in their diet along with plant foods. They avoid meat, poultry, fish, and eggs but consume foods like milk, cheese, yogurt, and other dairy products.

- Ovo-Vegetarian: Ovo-vegetarians exclude dairy products but include eggs in their diet along with plant foods. They avoid meat, poultry, fish, and dairy but consume eggs as a source of animal protein.

- Lacto-Ovo-Vegetarian: Lacto-ovo-vegetarians include both dairy products and eggs in their diet along with plant foods.

They exclude meat, poultry, and fish but consume dairy products and eggs.

These variations offer flexibility in meeting individual dietary preferences, cultural practices, and nutritional needs while still emphasizing plant-based foods as the foundation of the diet.

Vegetarian diets can be nutritionally balanced and provide a wide range of nutrients when planned appropriately. However, it is important for vegetarians, especially vegans and those who exclude certain food groups, to ensure they are meeting their nutritional requirements, including protein, iron, vitamin B12, calcium, and omega-3 fatty acids. Seeking guidance from a healthcare professional or registered dietitian can help vegetarians optimize their diet for adequate nutrient intake.

3. Flexitarian or Semi-Vegetarian Diet

This diet is primarily plant-based such as fruits, vegetables, whole grains, legumes, nuts, and seeds. These foods provide a rich array of nutrients, fiber, and antioxidants.

However, unlike strict vegetarians or vegans, flexitarians may include animal protein sources on occasion. The amount and frequency of meat, poultry, or fish consumption can vary depending on individual preferences and dietary goals. Some flexitarians may choose to have a meatless day or two each week, while others may include small portions of animal protein in their meals a few times per week.

The flexitarian approach allows individuals to enjoy the benefits of plant-based eating while still accommodating personal preferences and cultural considerations. It can provide the opportunity to explore a wider variety of foods and flavors while reducing the overall intake of animal products.

As with any diet, it's important for flexitarians to focus on nutrient balance and ensure they are meeting their nutritional needs. Emphasizing a variety of plant-based foods and making informed choices when consuming animal products can help maintain a healthful and balanced flexitarian diet.

4. Pescatarian Diet

A pescatarian diet is a primarily plant-based eating pattern that includes fish and seafood while excluding other types of meat, such as poultry, beef, pork, and other land animals. Pescatarians derive the majority of their nutrition from plant sources, like fruits, vegetables, whole grains, legumes, nuts, and seeds, while incorporating fish and seafood as their primary animal protein sources.

Fish and seafood provide important nutrients such as omega-3 fatty acids, high-quality protein, vitamins (such as vitamin D and vitamin B12), and minerals (such as iodine and selenium). Omega-3 fatty acids, in particular, are known for their heart-healthy benefits and are abundant in fatty fish like salmon, mackerel, sardines, and trout.

By including fish and seafood, pescatarians can potentially benefit from the nutrients found in these animal-derived foods while still adhering to a plant-centered approach. This dietary choice can offer a wide range of flavors and culinary options while reducing the consumption of other types of meat.

It's important for pescatarians to make informed choices about the types of fish and seafood they consume, as some species may be high in mercury or other contaminants. Opting for sustainable and low-mercury options, such as wild-caught salmon or sardines, can help minimize potential risks.

As with any diet, ensuring a balanced intake of nutrients is essential. Pescatarians should focus on incorporating a variety of plant-based foods, including whole grains, legumes, fruits, and vegetables, to obtain essential vitamins, minerals, and fiber. Consulting with a healthcare professional or registered dietitian can provide personalized guidance to ensure nutritional needs are met while following a pescatarian diet.

Plant-based diets emphasize the consumption of whole, minimally processed foods that are rich in nutrients, fiber, and antioxidants. They typically include a variety of fruits, vegetables, whole grains, legumes, nuts, and seeds. These diets can be customized based on individual preferences and nutritional needs.

The benefits of plant-based diets include lower risks of chronic diseases such as heart disease, diabetes, certain cancers, and obesity. They are also associated with improved nutrient intake, weight management, and overall health.

It's important to note that while plant-based diets can be nutritionally adequate, attention should be given to certain nutrients that may be lacking, such as vitamin B12, iron, calcium, and omega-3 fatty acids. Consulting with a healthcare professional or a registered dietitian can provide personalized guidance to ensure proper nutrient balance when following a plant-based diet.

Research on Plant-Based Diets in Disease Reversal

Plant-based diets have been the subject of extensive research regarding their potential to prevent and even reverse certain chronic diseases. Numerous studies have shown that adopting a plant-based eating pattern, particularly one that is low in saturated fats and rich in fruits, vegetables, whole grains, and legumes, can significantly reduce the risk of heart disease.

These diets have been associated with lower cholesterol levels, blood pressure, and body weight, all of which are key factors in heart health. Furthermore, the high fiber and antioxidant content of plant-based diets may contribute to their positive impact on cardiovascular health. A systematic review and meta-analysis found that vegetarian diets were associated with improved glycemic control in individuals with diabetes, suggesting that plant-based diets may have benefits for managing type 2 diabetes as well.

In addition to heart disease and diabetes, plant-based diets have also been studied in the context of obesity. The emphasis on nutrient-dense, low-calorie foods and the high fiber content of plant-based diets can contribute to weight loss and weight management. The lower energy density of plant-based foods, combined with their satiating effect, may help individuals maintain a healthier body weight. Furthermore, plant-based diets have been shown to influence gut microbiota composition, which may play a role in weight regulation and metabolic health.

While research on the relationship between plant-based diets and cancer prevention is ongoing, some studies have suggested a potential protective effect. Plant-based diets, rich in antioxidants, fiber, and phytochemicals, may help reduce the risk of certain types of cancer, such as colorectal and breast cancer. Additionally, maintaining a healthy body weight through plant-based diets may further contribute to a lower risk of developing cancer.

It is important to note that individual dietary needs and preferences can vary, and adopting a plant-based diet should be done in consultation with healthcare professionals or registered dietitians. They can provide personalized guidance to ensure that the diet is nutritionally balanced and suitable for specific health conditions. Nonetheless, the existing body of research supports the notion that plant-based diets have the potential to be a powerful tool in disease prevention and management.

Tips for Adopting a Plant-Based Lifestyle

Adopting a plant-based lifestyle can be a positive step towards improving your health and promoting sustainability. Here are some tips to help you transition to a plant-based diet:

1. Start gradually

Instead of making sudden and drastic changes, consider easing into a plant-based lifestyle by gradually incorporating more plant-based meals into your diet. Begin with one or two meatless days per week and gradually increase the number of plant-based meals over time.

2. Focus on whole, unprocessed foods

Emphasize whole grains, fruits, vegetables, legumes, nuts, and seeds as the foundation of your diet. These foods provide essential nutrients and fiber while minimizing added sugars, unhealthy fats, and artificial ingredients.

3. Experiment with plant-based alternatives

Explore a variety of plant-based alternatives to animal products, such as tofu, tempeh, seitan, and plant-based milk. These options can add variety and texture to your meals and help you transition away from animal-based products.

4. Educate yourself on plant-based nutrition

Ensure that you're meeting your nutritional needs by familiarizing yourself with plant-based sources of protein, iron, calcium, omega-3 fatty acids, and other essential nutrients. Consider consulting a registered dietitian to develop a well-balanced plant-based meal plan tailored to your individual needs.

5. Get creative with cooking

Explore new recipes and cooking techniques to make your plant-based meals flavorful and enjoyable. Experiment with herbs, spices, and different cooking methods to enhance the taste and texture of plant-based ingredients.

6. Plan and prepare meals in advance

Take time to plan your meals and snacks for the week ahead. This will help you stay organized, ensure you have plant-based options readily available, and reduce the likelihood of resorting to less healthy choices.

7. Find support and inspiration

Connect with others who follow a plant-based lifestyle for support and recipe ideas. Join online communities, participate in plant-based challenges, or attend local events focused on plant-based living.

8. Be mindful of nutrient balance

Pay attention to your nutrient intake, particularly vitamins B12 and D, iron, calcium, and omega-3 fatty acids. Consider supplements or fortified foods to meet your nutritional needs, if necessary.

9. Enjoy the process

Approach your plant-based journey with a sense of curiosity and enjoyment. Discover new flavors, embrace the variety of plant-based foods, and appreciate the positive impact your choices have on your health and the environment.

Remember, everyone's journey towards a plant-based lifestyle is unique. It's important to listen to your body, make adjustments as needed, and prioritize your overall well-being.

Chapter 7

Gut Health and Disease Prevention

Gut health plays a crucial role in disease prevention by influencing various aspects of our overall well-being. The gut microbiota, which consists of trillions of microorganisms living in our intestines, has a profound impact on our immune system, digestion, inflammation levels, mental health, and disease risk.

A healthy gut microbiota helps maintain a strong immune system, defending against infections and reducing the risk of autoimmune disorders and allergies. It supports proper digestion and nutrient absorption, promoting digestive health and reducing the risk of gastrointestinal disorders. Additionally, a balanced gut microbiota helps regulate inflammation throughout the body, lowering the risk of chronic diseases like cardiovascular disease, diabetes, and certain cancers.

The gut-brain axis highlights the connection between the gut and the brain, indicating that a healthy gut can contribute to good mental health and cognitive function. By nourishing our gut microbiota through a diverse and fiber-rich diet, we can support gut health and potentially reduce the risk of chronic diseases such as obesity, cardiovascular disease, and certain cancers.

While the research on gut health and disease prevention is ongoing, adopting a lifestyle that promotes a healthy gut, including a diet rich in fruits, vegetables, whole grains, and probiotic-rich foods, can have a positive impact on our overall health and well-being. It is always beneficial to consult with healthcare professionals or registered dietitians for personalized guidance on optimizing gut health and disease prevention.

Understanding the Gut Microbiome and Its Role in Health

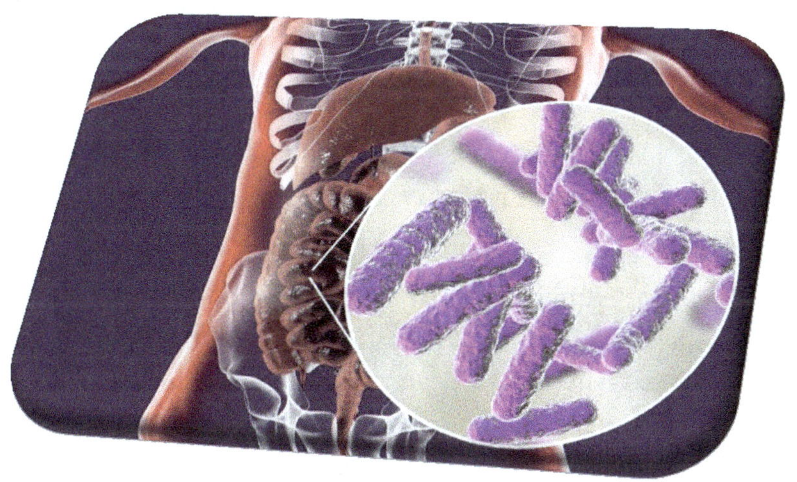

The gut microbiome refers to the collection of microorganisms, including bacteria, viruses, fungi, and other microbes, that reside in the gastrointestinal tract, particularly the large intestine. It is a complex and diverse ecosystem that plays a crucial role in our overall health and well-being.

The gut microbiome is unique to each individual, and its composition can be influenced by various factors such as genetics, diet, lifestyle, medications, and environmental exposures. It is estimated that the gut microbiome consists of trillions of microorganisms, with thousands of different species.

The microorganisms in the gut microbiome have important functions that contribute to our health.

- They help with the digestion and metabolism of dietary components that our own body cannot break down, such as certain fibers.

- They produce essential nutrients like vitamins B and K. They interact with our immune system, influencing immune responses and defense against pathogens.

- They also play a role in maintaining the integrity of the intestinal barrier and preventing the colonization of harmful bacteria.

Research on the gut microbiome has expanded our understanding of its impact on various aspects of health, including digestion, immune function, metabolism, mental health, and disease risk. Imbalances or disruptions in the gut microbiome, known as dysbiosis, have been associated with a range of health conditions, including gastrointestinal disorders, obesity, autoimmune diseases, and mental health disorders.

Studying the gut microbiome and its interactions with our body is an active area of research, and ongoing advancements continue to deepen our understanding of its significance.

Here are some of the major microorganisms commonly found in the gut:

1. Bacteria

Bacteria are the most abundant microorganisms in the gut microbiome. Some of the prominent bacterial phyla include:

- Firmicutes: This phylum includes bacteria like *Lactobacillus*, *Clostridium*, and *Ruminococcus*.

- Bacteroidetes: This phylum includes bacteria like *Bacteroides* and *Prevotella*.

- Actinobacteria: This phylum includes bacteria like *Bifidobacterium* and *Collinsella*.

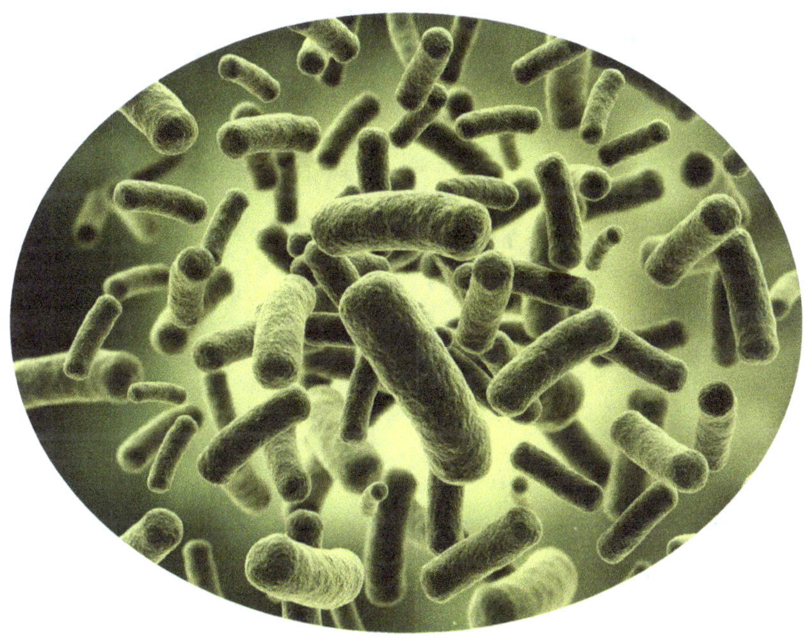

2. Viruses

Viruses that reside in the gut are mainly bacteriophages, which are viruses that infect bacteria. These viruses can have a significant impact on the composition and function of the gut microbiome. Examples are CrAssphage, PhiX174, T4 phage and Lambda phage.

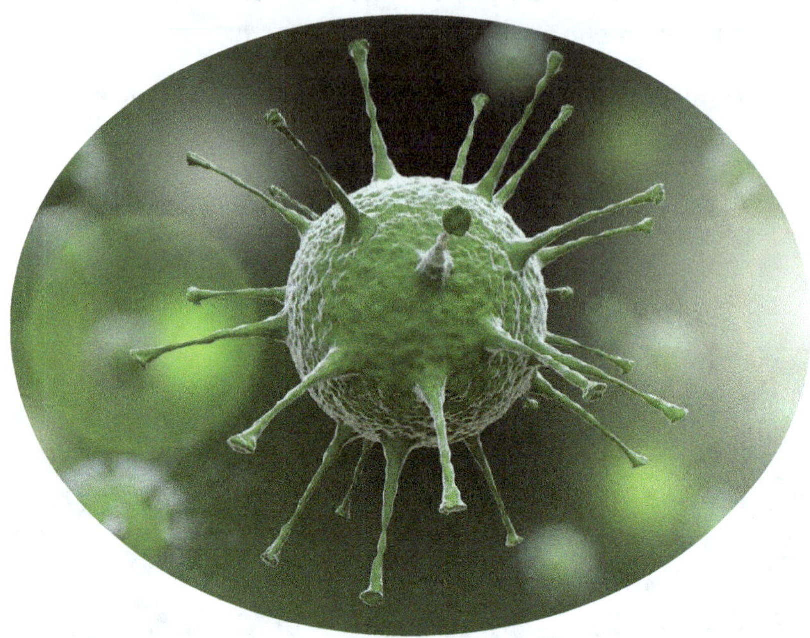

3. Fungi

Fungi found in the gut include various species of yeasts and molds. *Candida* and *Saccharomyces* are examples of fungal genera that can be present in the gut microbiome.

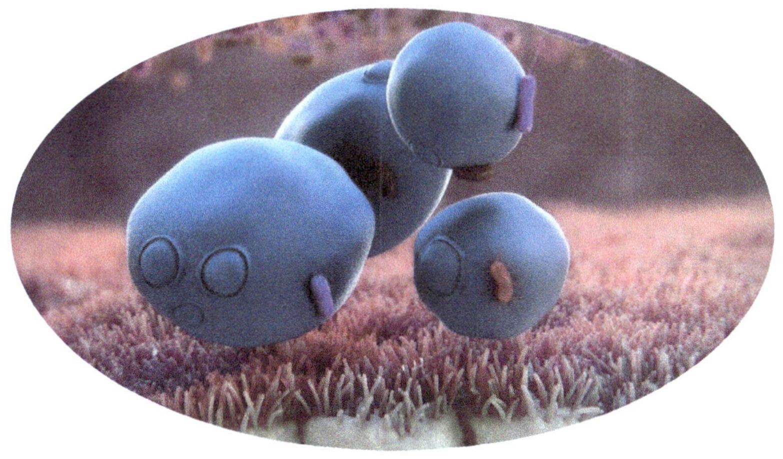

4. Archaea

Archaea are a group of single-celled microorganisms that are genetically distinct from bacteria. *Methanobrevibacter* is an example of an archaeal genus commonly found in the gut.

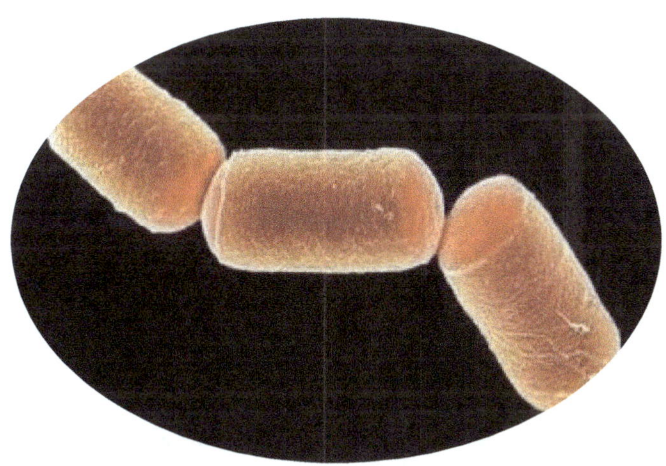

Microorganisms in the gut, collectively known as the gut microbiota or gut microbiome, play various essential roles in maintaining overall health and contributing to numerous physiological processes.

Here are some key roles of microbiome in the gut:

1. Digestion and Nutrient Metabolism

The gut microbiota helps in the digestion and breakdown of complex carbohydrates, dietary fibers, and other components of our diet that our own body cannot fully digest. They produce enzymes that break down these substances into simpler forms, facilitating nutrient absorption and energy production. For example, certain gut bacteria ferment dietary fibers and produce short-chain fatty acids, which serve as an energy source for our intestinal cells.

2. Immune System Regulation

The gut microbiota interacts closely with our immune system, playing a vital role in immune system development and function. They help educate and regulate the immune system, contributing to immune tolerance and preventing inappropriate immune responses. The presence of beneficial gut bacteria can help suppress harmful pathogens, while an imbalance in the gut microbiota can lead to immune dysregulation and increased susceptibility to infections and autoimmune disorders.

3. Synthesis of Vitamins and Nutrients

Certain gut bacteria have the ability to synthesize vitamins, such as vitamin K and certain B vitamins (e.g., biotin and folate). They also aid in the absorption of minerals like magnesium and calcium.

The production of these essential nutrients by the gut microbiota enhances our overall nutritional status.

4. Protection Against Pathogens

The gut microbiota acts as a barrier against harmful bacteria and pathogens. By colonizing the gut lining and competing for resources, beneficial bacteria can prevent the growth and colonization of harmful microorganisms. They can also produce antimicrobial substances that inhibit the growth of pathogens and support a healthy gut environment.

5. Metabolic Regulation

Emerging evidence suggests that the gut microbiota can influence metabolic processes, including energy balance, glucose metabolism, and lipid metabolism. Imbalances in the gut microbiota, such as a decrease in microbial diversity or an overgrowth of certain harmful bacteria, have been associated with metabolic disorders like obesity and type 2 diabetes.

It's important to note that the roles and functions of the gut microbiota are still an active area of research, and our understanding of their complexity is continuously evolving. The composition and function of the gut microbiota can be influenced by various factors, including diet, lifestyle, medications, and environmental exposures. Maintaining a diverse and balanced gut microbiota through a healthy diet and lifestyle is crucial for overall health and well-being.

Foods that Promote a Healthy Gut Microbiome

A healthy gut microbiome thrives on a diverse range of nutrients and dietary fibers. Including the following foods in your diet can promote a healthy gut microbiome:

1. Fiber-rich Foods

Foods high in fiber are excellent for promoting a healthy gut microbiome. They include fruits, vegetables, whole grains, legumes, nuts, and seeds. Fiber acts as a prebiotic, providing nourishment to beneficial gut bacteria and promoting their growth.

2. Fermented Foods

Fermented foods are rich in beneficial bacteria known as probiotics, which can help improve gut health. Examples include yogurt, kefir, sauerkraut, kimchi, tempeh, and miso. These foods introduce live microorganisms into the gut, contributing to a diverse and healthy gut microbiome.

3. Prebiotic Foods

Prebiotics are non-digestible fibers that serve as food for beneficial gut bacteria. They include foods like onions, garlic, leeks, asparagus, bananas, artichokes, and whole grains. Consuming prebiotic-rich foods can help nourish and support the growth of beneficial gut bacteria.

4. Polyphenol-rich Foods

Polyphenols are plant compounds with antioxidant properties that can benefit the gut microbiome. Foods rich in polyphenols include berries, grapes, green tea, cocoa, nuts, and spices like turmeric and cinnamon. Polyphenols can help modulate the gut microbiota composition and promote a healthy microbial balance.

5. Omega-3 Fatty Acid Sources

Foods rich in omega-3 fatty acids, such as fatty fish (salmon, mackerel), chia seeds, flaxseeds, and walnuts, can have a positive impact on gut health. Omega-3 fatty acids help reduce gut inflammation and support the growth of beneficial bacteria.

6. Diversity of Plant-based Foods

Incorporating a wide variety of plant-based foods in your diet is essential for a healthy gut microbiome. Aim to include different types of fruits, vegetables, whole grains, legumes, nuts, and seeds to provide a broad spectrum of nutrients and fibers for your gut microbiota.

Remember that promoting a healthy gut microbiome is not just about individual foods but also about adopting a balanced and varied diet. It's best to consult with a healthcare professional or registered dietitian for personalized dietary recommendations to support your gut health.

Gut Health and Disease Reversal: Recent Scientific Findings

Scientific research has increasingly highlighted the critical role of gut health in disease prevention and even disease reversal. Here are some recent scientific findings linking gut health to disease:

1. Inflammatory Bowel Disease (IBD)

Studies have shown that alterations in the gut microbiota composition and function contribute to the development and progression of IBD, including Crohn's disease and ulcerative colitis. Restoring a healthy gut microbiota through interventions like fecal microbiota transplantation (FMT) or targeted probiotic and prebiotic therapies has shown promise in reducing inflammation and improving symptoms in IBD patients.

2. Obesity and Metabolic Disorders

Imbalances in the gut microbiota, characterized by reduced microbial diversity and an overgrowth of certain bacterial species, have been associated with obesity and metabolic disorders such as insulin resistance and type 2 diabetes. Research suggests that modulating the gut microbiota through dietary interventions, such as increased fiber intake and specific probiotic supplementation, may help improve metabolic health and promote weight loss.

3. Mental Health Disorders

The gut-brain axis, a bidirectional communication system between the gut and the brain, plays a crucial role in mental health. Alterations in the gut microbiota have been linked to mental health disorders, including anxiety and depression. Emerging evidence suggests that interventions targeting the gut microbiota, such as probiotic supplementation and dietary changes, may have a positive impact on mental health outcomes.

4. Cardiovascular Health

The gut microbiota can influence cardiovascular health through various mechanisms, including the production of metabolites that affect lipid metabolism, inflammation, and blood pressure regulation. Recent studies have identified specific gut microbial signatures associated with cardiovascular disease. Modulating the gut microbiota through dietary interventions, such as increasing fiber intake and consuming polyphenol-rich foods, may have potential benefits for cardiovascular health.

5. Autoimmune Diseases

Autoimmune diseases, such as rheumatoid arthritis and multiple sclerosis, have been linked to dysregulation of the gut microbiota and increased intestinal permeability ("leaky gut"). Research suggests that interventions targeting gut health, including probiotics, prebiotics, and dietary modifications, may help modulate immune responses and improve symptoms in autoimmune diseases.

These findings highlight the significance of gut health in disease prevention and potential disease reversal. While the field of gut microbiome research is still evolving, these scientific insights offer promising avenues for the development of targeted interventions to improve health outcomes. It's important to note that further research is needed to fully understand the complex interactions between the gut microbiota, diet, and specific diseases, and to identify optimal strategies for gut health optimization.

Chapter 8

The Role of Specific Foods in Disease Prevention and Reversal

Food and health are inextricably linked, and recent research has shown the important role that some foods can play in disease prevention and even reversal. Scientific research indicates that some dietary decisions can have a significant impact on our health, even if no one meal can offer total immunity from all diseases. We will examine the significance of specific foods in disease avoidance and reversal, highlighting the expanding knowledge of the relationship between nutrition and general health. People may be able to lower their risk of contracting numerous diseases and improve their overall quality of life by making informed eating decisions.

They include the followings:

Berries: Nature's Disease-Fighting Gems

Berries are often hailed as nature's disease-fighting gems due to their impressive nutritional profiles and numerous health benefits. These small, colorful fruits are packed with vitamins, minerals, antioxidants, and other bioactive compounds that contribute to their disease-fighting properties. Here are some reasons why berries are considered beneficial for health:

1. Antioxidant Power

Berries are rich in antioxidants, such as anthocyanins, flavonols, and vitamin C. These compounds help neutralize harmful free radicals in the body, which can prevent oxidative stress and damage to cells. By reducing oxidative stress, berries may help lower the risk of chronic diseases like heart disease, cancer, and neurodegenerative disorders.

2. Anti-Inflammatory Effects

Chronic inflammation is associated with various diseases, including heart disease, diabetes, and certain types of cancer. Berries contain anti-inflammatory compounds that can help reduce inflammation in the body. For instance, anthocyanins found in berries have been shown to inhibit inflammation and provide protective effects.

3. Heart Health

Berries, particularly blueberries and strawberries, have been linked to heart health benefits. Their high content of antioxidants, fiber, and polyphenols may contribute to reducing the risk of heart disease. Regular berry consumption has been associated with improved blood pressure, increased levels of good cholesterol (HDL), and reduced oxidation of LDL (bad) cholesterol.

4. Cognitive Function

Several studies have suggested that the consumption of berries may support brain health and improve cognitive function. The antioxidants and other bioactive compounds in berries have been shown to protect the brain from oxidative stress and inflammation, potentially reducing the risk of age-related cognitive decline and neurodegenerative disorders like Alzheimer's disease

5. Blood Sugar Regulation

Berries generally have a low glycemic index, meaning they do not cause a rapid increase in blood sugar levels. This characteristic, along with their fiber content, may help regulate blood sugar levels and improve insulin sensitivity. This makes berries a good choice for individuals with diabetes or those aiming to prevent it.

6. Digestive Health

Berries are a good source of dietary fiber, which promotes healthy digestion. Fiber helps regulate bowel movements, prevent constipation, and supports a healthy gut microbiome. Consuming a variety of berries can contribute to overall digestive health.

7. Cancer Prevention

While further research is needed, some studies suggest that the antioxidants and other bioactive compounds in berries may have anti-cancer properties. These compounds can help protect cells from DNA damage, inhibit the growth of cancer cells, and reduce inflammation associated with certain types of cancer.

It's important to note that while berries offer various health benefits, they should be part of a balanced diet that includes a variety of fruits, vegetables, whole grains, lean proteins, and other nutrient-rich foods. Incorporating a wide range of colorful fruits and vegetables into your diet is key to obtaining a diverse array of beneficial compounds for optimal health.

Cruciferous Vegetables: Harnessing their Anti-Cancer Properties

Cruciferous vegetables, which belong to the Brassicaceae family, are known for their unique combination of flavors, textures, and most importantly, their potent anti-cancer properties. These vegetables are packed with essential nutrients, fiber, and a variety of bioactive compounds that have been extensively studied for their potential to prevent and fight cancer. Here's an overview of the key reasons why cruciferous vegetables are considered beneficial in harnessing their anti-cancer properties:

1. Sulforaphane and Indole-3-Carbinol

Cruciferous vegetables, such as broccoli, cabbage, cauliflower, kale, Brussels sprouts, and bok choy, contain compounds called sulforaphane and indole-3-carbinol. These compounds have been shown to have anti-cancer effects by activating detoxification enzymes, inhibiting the growth of cancer cells, and promoting their apoptosis (programmed cell death).

2. Antioxidant and Anti-Inflammatory Properties

Cruciferous vegetables are rich in antioxidants, including vitamins C and E, beta-carotene, and various flavonoids. These antioxidants help neutralize harmful free radicals and reduce oxidative stress in the body, which is associated with cancer development. Additionally, the high fiber content of these vegetables promotes healthy digestion and reduces chronic inflammation, which can contribute to cancer progression.

3. Detoxification Support

Certain compounds in cruciferous vegetables, particularly broccoli sprouts, have been found to enhance the body's detoxification processes. Sulforaphane, in particular, activates a specific pathway in the body called the Nrf2 pathway, which helps remove harmful toxins and carcinogens, reducing the risk of cancer.

4. Hormone Regulation

Some cruciferous vegetables, such as broccoli and cabbage, contain compounds that can help regulate hormones in the body. For example, indole-3-carbinol has been shown to convert excess estrogen into a less potent form, potentially reducing the risk of hormone-related cancers, such as breast and prostate cancer.

5. Anti-Angiogenesis Effects

Cruciferous vegetables may also exhibit anti-angiogenesis properties. Angiogenesis is the process of forming new blood vessels to supply nutrients to growing tumors. Certain compounds in cruciferous vegetables, such as sulforaphane, have been found to inhibit angiogenesis, thereby potentially limiting the blood supply to cancer cells and impeding their growth.

6. Gut Microbiome Health

Cruciferous vegetables contain dietary fiber that acts as a prebiotic, promoting the growth of beneficial bacteria in the gut. A healthy gut microbiome is increasingly recognized as important for overall health, including cancer prevention. Some studies suggest that the metabolites produced by gut bacteria from cruciferous vegetable consumption may have anti-cancer effects.

It's worth noting that while cruciferous vegetables offer potential anti-cancer benefits, individual responses may vary, and they should be part of a well-balanced diet that includes a variety of fruits, vegetables, whole grains, lean proteins, and healthy fats. Additionally, cooking methods can affect the bioavailability of the beneficial compounds, so it's advisable to use gentle cooking techniques like steaming or stir-frying to retain their nutritional value.

Whole Grains: Promoting Heart Health and Diabetes Prevention

Whole grains are an important component of a healthy diet and are known for their potential to promote heart health and help prevent diabetes. Unlike refined grains, which have had their bran and germ removed, whole grains retain these nutritious components, providing a rich source of fiber, vitamins, minerals, and phytochemicals. Here are the key ways in which whole grains contribute to heart health and diabetes prevention:

1. Fiber Content

Whole grains are an excellent source of dietary fiber, which offers several benefits for heart health and diabetes prevention. Fiber helps regulate blood sugar levels by slowing down the absorption of glucose and improving insulin sensitivity. It also aids in maintaining a healthy body weight and reducing the risk of developing type 2 diabetes.

2. Lower Risk of Heart Disease

Consuming whole grains has been associated with a reduced risk of heart disease. The fiber, antioxidants, and phytochemicals in whole grains contribute to this protective effect. High-fiber diets have been linked to lower levels of LDL (bad) cholesterol, improved blood pressure, and reduced inflammation, all of which are risk factors for heart disease.

3. Blood Pressure Management

Whole grains, especially those rich in magnesium, such as whole wheat, brown rice, and quinoa, can help regulate blood pressure. Magnesium has been shown to relax blood vessels, leading to improved blood flow and lower blood pressure levels.

4. Nutrient Content

Whole grains are a good source of essential nutrients, including B vitamins, vitamin E, magnesium, zinc, and iron. These nutrients are important for overall heart health and help support the body's metabolic processes. By incorporating whole grains into your diet, you can ensure you're obtaining these essential nutrients.

5. Weight Management

Whole grains, due to their fiber content, provide a greater feeling of fullness and can help manage weight. They take longer to digest, reducing the likelihood of overeating and aiding in weight control. Maintaining a healthy weight is crucial for reducing the risk of developing type 2 diabetes and managing heart health.

6. Glycemic Control

Whole grains have a lower glycemic index compared to refined grains. The glycemic index measures how quickly a food raises blood sugar levels. Whole grains release glucose more slowly, resulting in a more gradual rise in blood sugar. This is beneficial for individuals with diabetes or those at risk of developing the condition.

7. Source of Antioxidants

Whole grains contain various antioxidants, including phenolic compounds and lignans, which have been associated with a reduced risk of heart disease. These antioxidants help protect against oxidative stress and inflammation, which are underlying factors in the development of cardiovascular diseases.

To reap the benefits of whole grains, it's recommended to choose minimally processed options such as whole wheat, brown rice, oats, quinoa, and barley. Incorporating a variety of whole grains into your meals, such as whole grain bread, pasta, and cereals, can help maximize their health-promoting effects.

Nuts and Seeds: Nutritional Powerhouses for Disease Reversal

Nuts and seeds are indeed nutritional powerhouses that offer a range of health benefits and have been associated with disease prevention and even reversal in some cases. They are rich in healthy fats, protein, fiber, vitamins, minerals, and various bioactive compounds. Here are some reasons why nuts and seeds are considered beneficial for disease reversal and overall health:

1. Heart Health

Nuts and seeds, including almonds, walnuts, flaxseeds, chia seeds, and hemp seeds, have been shown to have a positive impact on heart health. They are high in monounsaturated and polyunsaturated fats, including omega-3 fatty acids, which can help lower LDL (bad) cholesterol levels, reduce inflammation, and improve overall lipid profiles. Regular consumption of nuts and seeds has been associated with a reduced risk of heart disease and cardiovascular events.

2. Diabetes Management

Despite their relatively high fat content, nuts and seeds have a low glycemic index and can be part of a healthy diet for individuals with diabetes. They provide a good source of protein, healthy fats, and fiber, which can help regulate blood sugar levels, improve insulin sensitivity, and reduce the risk of developing type 2 diabetes.

3. Weight Management

Despite being energy-dense, nuts and seeds can be beneficial for weight management. Their combination of protein, fiber, and healthy fats can increase satiety and reduce appetite, potentially leading to decreased calorie intake. Incorporating moderate portions of nuts and seeds into a balanced diet can support healthy weight management.

4. Nutrient Density

Nuts and seeds are rich in essential nutrients, including vitamin E, magnesium, potassium, calcium, and various B vitamins. These nutrients are important for overall health, immune function, energy production, and maintaining healthy bones and muscles.

5. Antioxidant and Anti-Inflammatory Properties

Nuts and seeds contain antioxidants, such as vitamin E and polyphenols, which can help reduce oxidative stress and inflammation in the body. Chronic inflammation and oxidative stress are underlying factors in many chronic diseases, including heart disease, diabetes, and certain types of cancer.

6. Gut Health

Certain nuts and seeds, such as almonds and flaxseeds, provide prebiotic fibers that support the growth of beneficial gut bacteria. A healthy gut microbiome is important for digestive health, nutrient absorption, immune function, and even mental well-being.

7. Cancer Prevention

Although more research is needed, some studies suggest that nuts and seeds may play a role in reducing the risk of certain types of cancer.

They contain various bioactive compounds, including phytosterols, lignans, and flavonoids, which have shown potential anti-cancer properties by inhibiting tumor growth and reducing inflammation.

It's important to consume nuts and seeds in moderation as they are energy-dense. A handful of nuts or a tablespoon of seeds per day is generally recommended as a healthy portion size. It's also advisable to choose unsalted varieties to avoid excessive sodium intake. Adding nuts and seeds to salads, yogurt, smoothies, or enjoying them as a snack can be a delicious and nutritious way to incorporate them into your diet.

Chapter 9

Mindful Eating and Disease Prevention

Mindful eating is a practice that involves being fully present and attentive while eating, without judgment. By slowing down and paying attention to the physical and emotional experience of eating, individuals can prevent certain diseases and improve their overall well-being. It helps individuals become more aware of their hunger and fullness cues, leading to better portion control and reduced risk of overeating or mindless snacking. By making conscious food choices and savoring each bite, mindful eating promotes a balanced and nutrient-dense diet, which is essential for disease prevention.

Practicing mindful eating can also have a positive impact on emotional eating and stress-related behaviors. By developing a non-judgmental attitude towards food and tuning into their body's needs, individuals can reduce the reliance on food as a coping mechanism and better manage emotional triggers. This can help prevent the development of chronic diseases associated with emotional eating, such as obesity and cardiovascular conditions. Mindful eating encourages individuals to cultivate a healthier relationship with food, leading to improved mental and emotional well-being.

Incorporating mindful eating into daily routines can contribute to long-term health by fostering a sense of self-awareness and self-care. By being fully present during meals, individuals can enhance the enjoyment and satisfaction derived from eating, reducing the desire for excessive or unhealthy foods. This practice promotes mindful food choices, encouraging individuals to prioritize nutrient-dense options and limit the consumption of processed and sugary foods. Overall, mindful eating supports disease prevention by promoting mindful food choices, portion control, emotional well-being, and a healthier relationship with food.

The Mind-Body Connection: How Mindful Eating Impacts Health

The mind-body connection refers to the interplay between our mental and emotional state and its influence on our physical health. Mindful eating is an approach that emphasizes awareness and presence during the eating experience, promoting a deeper connection between the mind and body. It involves paying attention to the sensory aspects of eating, such as the taste, smell, and texture of food, as well as being aware of hunger and fullness cues.

Here's how mindful eating can impact health:

1. Improved Digestion

When we eat mindfully, we tend to slow down and savor our food. This allows for better digestion as our bodies can focus on breaking down and absorbing nutrients more effectively. Chewing food thoroughly, being present during meals, and paying attention to the process of eating can help reduce digestive issues like bloating and discomfort.

2. Weight Management

Mindful eating can be a powerful tool for weight management. By paying attention to hunger and fullness cues, we become more attuned to our body's needs and can better regulate portion sizes. Mindful eating also helps us distinguish between true physical hunger and emotional or mindless eating, reducing the likelihood of overeating.

3. Enhanced Satisfaction and Enjoyment

When we eat mindfully, we fully engage with the eating experience. By focusing on the taste, texture, and aroma of our food, we can derive more pleasure and satisfaction from what we eat. This can lead to a greater sense of enjoyment and reduce the tendency to seek satisfaction from excessive or unhealthy food choices.

4. Increased Awareness of Food Choices

Mindful eating encourages self-awareness and reflection on our food choices. By paying attention to how different foods make us feel physically and emotionally, we can make more conscious and nourishing choices that support our overall health and well-being.

5. Emotional Regulation

Mindful eating involves being present with our thoughts, feelings, and emotions that arise during meals. This heightened awareness allows us to observe and better understand our relationship with food. It can help us identify emotional triggers for overeating or unhealthy eating patterns, leading to improved emotional regulation and a healthier approach to food.

6. Stress Reduction

Mindful eating can be a form of stress management. Taking the time to sit down, focus on our food, and create a calm eating environment can help reduce stress levels. When we eat in a relaxed state, our bodies are better able to digest food and absorb nutrients effectively.

7. Connection to Body Signals

By practicing mindful eating, we learn to listen to our body's signals of hunger, fullness, and satisfaction. This connection to our body's needs can help us make informed decisions about when and what to eat, promoting a balanced and intuitive approach to eating.

Incorporating mindfulness into meals can be as simple as eating without distractions, taking time to appreciate the flavors and textures of the food, and checking in with your body's hunger and fullness cues. Cultivating a mindful eating practice can contribute to a healthier relationship with food and positively impact overall health and well-being.

Strategies for Practicing Mindful Eating

Practicing mindful eating involves bringing a sense of awareness, attention, and non-judgment to the entire eating experience. Here are some strategies to help you cultivate mindful eating habits:

1. Slow Down

Take your time to eat and savor each bite. Chew your food thoroughly and fully experience the flavors and textures.

Putting your utensils down between bites can help you eat at a more leisurely pace.

2. Remove Distractions

Minimize distractions during meals by turning off the TV, putting away electronic devices, and finding a quiet space to eat. This allows you to focus solely on the eating experience and be fully present.

3. Engage Your Senses

Pay attention to the sensory aspects of eating. Notice the colors, smells, textures, and flavors of your food. Take time to appreciate the visual appeal and aroma before taking your first bite.

4. Listen to Your Body

Tune in to your body's hunger and fullness cues. Before eating, ask yourself how hungry you are on a scale from 1 to 10. During the meal, periodically check in with yourself to assess your level of fullness. Eat until you are satisfied, not overly stuffed.

5. Practice Non-Judgment

Approach eating with a non-judgmental mindset. Avoid labeling foods as "good" or "bad." Instead, focus on nourishing your body and making choices that support your well-being. Be kind to yourself and cultivate self-compassion around your eating habits.

6. Be Mindful of Emotional Eating

Notice any emotional triggers that may be influencing your eating habits. Are you eating out of boredom, stress, or other emotional states? Take a moment to pause and reflect on your emotions before reaching for food. Consider alternative ways to address emotional needs.

7. Portion Control

Pay attention to portion sizes and aim to eat mindfully even when enjoying indulgent foods. Choose smaller plates or bowls, and take the time to savor each bite, regardless of the food's caloric content.

8. Practice Gratitude

Before starting your meal, take a moment to express gratitude for the food you are about to eat. This can help cultivate a sense of appreciation and mindfulness towards the nourishment it provides.

9. Keep a Food Journal

Consider keeping a food journal to track your eating habits and patterns. This can help increase awareness of your eating behaviors, emotions, and triggers, allowing you to make more informed choices.

10. Seek Support

Joining a mindful eating group or seeking support from a registered dietitian or therapist who specializes in mindful eating can provide guidance, accountability, and a sense of community as you develop your mindful eating practice.

Remember, mindful eating is a skill that takes time and practice to develop. Start with small steps and be patient with yourself as you cultivate a more mindful relationship with food.

Mindful Eating for Disease Prevention and Reversal

Mindful eating can be a valuable approach for disease prevention and even reversal when combined with a balanced and nutritious diet. While it is not a cure or standalone treatment for diseases, practicing mindful eating can positively impact overall health and contribute to disease management.

Here's how mindful eating can support disease prevention and reversal:

1. Weight Management

Mindful eating helps promote a healthier relationship with food, reducing the likelihood of overeating and supporting weight management. Maintaining a healthy weight is crucial for preventing and managing various chronic conditions such as heart disease, type 2 diabetes, and certain types of cancer.

2. Blood Sugar Control

Mindful eating can support better blood sugar control, especially for individuals with diabetes or those at risk of developing the condition. By being aware of hunger and fullness cues, choosing balanced meals, and paying attention to the glycemic load of foods, mindful eating can help regulate blood sugar levels and improve insulin sensitivity.

3. Heart Health

Adopting a mindful eating approach encourages making healthier food choices and being aware of the impact of certain foods on heart health. By focusing on whole, unprocessed foods and being mindful of portion sizes, mindful eating supports heart health by promoting a balanced diet, managing weight, and reducing the intake of unhealthy fats and added sugars.

4. Digestive Health

Mindful eating involves taking the time to chew food thoroughly, savoring flavors, and being present during meals. This can aid digestion by facilitating better nutrient absorption and reducing digestive discomfort such as bloating or indigestion.

5. Emotional Eating

Mindful eating can help address emotional eating patterns, which are often linked to stress, anxiety, or other emotional triggers. By becoming more aware of emotional cues and using mindfulness techniques to manage emotions, individuals can develop healthier coping mechanisms and reduce reliance on food for emotional comfort.

6. Nutrient Intake

Mindful eating encourages a focus on the quality of food choices, which can lead to an increased intake of nutrient-dense foods. By being present and engaged with the eating experience, individuals are more likely to choose whole, unprocessed foods that provide essential nutrients for disease prevention and overall health.

7. Mind-Body Connection

Mindful eating fosters a deeper connection between the mind and body. By being present and paying attention to physical sensations, individuals can become more attuned to their body's needs and respond accordingly. This can contribute to a more intuitive and balanced approach to eating, supporting overall well-being.

It's important to note that mindful eating should be part of a comprehensive approach to disease prevention and management. It is recommended to work with healthcare professionals, such as registered dietitians or healthcare providers, to develop a personalized plan that takes into account specific dietary needs, medical conditions, and individual goals.

Chapter 10

Recipes for Health: Delicious and Nutritious Dishes

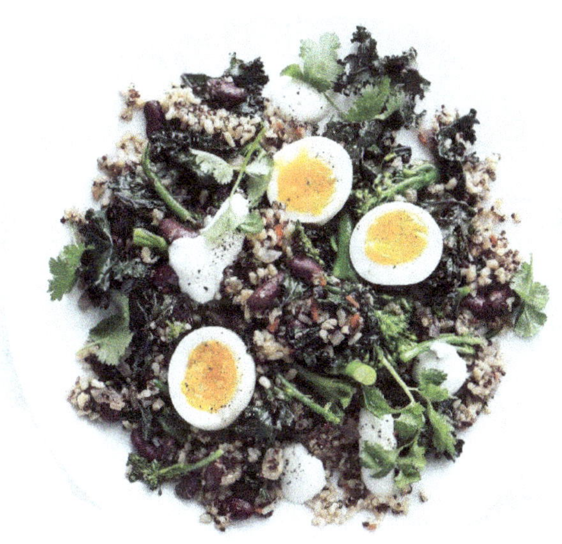

Recipes for health focus on creating dishes that are both delicious and packed with essential nutrients to support overall well-being. These recipes prioritize wholesome ingredients like fruits, vegetables, whole grains, lean proteins, and healthy fats. They often incorporate a variety of herbs, spices, and seasonings to enhance flavors without relying on excessive salt, sugar, or unhealthy additives.

From vibrant salads and nourishing soups to hearty main courses and guilt-free desserts, these recipes prioritize balance, incorporating a range of vitamins, minerals, antioxidants, and fiber. They emphasize using cooking methods that retain the nutritional value of the ingredients, such as steaming, grilling, baking, and sautéing.

Recipes for health are designed to promote disease prevention, support weight management, boost energy levels, and optimize overall health. They cater to various dietary preferences and restrictions, including vegetarian, vegan, gluten-free, and dairy-free options, ensuring that everyone can find delicious and nutritious dishes to suit their needs.

By embracing these recipes, individuals can enjoy the benefits of a well-rounded diet while indulging in mouthwatering flavors and textures. These dishes are not only satisfying but also contribute to long-term well-being and a healthier lifestyle.

Breakfast Ideas for Disease Prevention

Starting your day with a nutritious breakfast can contribute to disease prevention by providing essential nutrients and supporting overall health. Here are three breakfast ideas that promote disease prevention:

1. Overnight Chia Pudding

Ingredients:

- 2 tablespoons chia seeds

- 1 cup unsweetened almond milk (or any other milk of your choice)

- 1 tablespoon honey or maple syrup

- Fresh berries (e.g., blueberries, strawberries) for topping

- Nuts and seeds (e.g., almonds, pumpkin seeds) for topping

Instructions:

- In a jar or bowl, combine the chia seeds, almond milk, and honey or maple syrup. Stir well to evenly distribute the chia seeds.

- Cover the jar or bowl and refrigerate overnight or for at least 4 hours to allow the chia seeds to absorb the liquid and create a pudding-like consistency.

- In the morning, give the chia pudding a good stir. Top with fresh berries, nuts, and seeds for added flavor, texture, and nutrients.

- Enjoy the pudding chilled and start your day with a dose of fiber, omega-3 fatty acids, and antioxidants.

2. Veggie Omelette

Ingredients:

- 2 large eggs

- 1/4 cup diced bell peppers (any color)

- 1/4 cup diced tomatoes

- 1/4 cup chopped spinach

- 1/4 cup sliced mushrooms

- 1/4 cup diced onions

- Salt and pepper to taste

- 1 teaspoon olive oil or cooking spray

Instructions:

- In a bowl, beat the eggs and season with salt and pepper.

- Heat the olive oil or cooking spray in a non-stick skillet over medium heat.

- Add the onions, bell peppers, mushrooms, and tomatoes to the skillet. Sauté for a few minutes until the vegetables are tender.

- Add the chopped spinach to the skillet and cook for an additional minute until wilted.

- Pour the beaten eggs over the cooked vegetables, tilting the skillet to ensure even distribution.

- Allow the omelette to cook undisturbed for a few minutes until the edges are set.

- Gently flip the omelette to cook the other side, or fold it in half if desired.

- Cook for another minute until the eggs are fully cooked but still moist.

- Transfer the omelette to a plate and serve hot. Pair it with whole grain toast or a side of fresh fruit for a well-rounded breakfast.

3. Greek Yogurt Parfait

Ingredients:

- 1 cup Greek yogurt (plain or flavored)

- 1/4 cup granola (choose a low-sugar option)

- 1/4 cup mixed fresh berries (e.g., raspberries, blueberries)

- 1 tablespoon honey or maple syrup (optional)

Instructions:

- In a glass or bowl, layer the Greek yogurt, granola, and fresh berries.

- Drizzle with honey or maple syrup for added sweetness, if desired.

- Repeat the layers until all the ingredients are used, ending with a sprinkle of granola and a few berries on top.

- Enjoy the parfait immediately or refrigerate it for a refreshing and protein-packed breakfast.

These breakfast ideas provide a good balance of nutrients, including fiber, protein, vitamins, and antioxidants, which can support disease prevention and promote overall well-being.

Power-Packed Lunches and Snacks

Here are three power-packed lunch and snack ideas that provide nourishment and energy throughout the day:

1. Quinoa Salad with Roasted Vegetables

Ingredients:

- 1 cup cooked quinoa
- 1 cup mixed roasted vegetables (e.g., bell peppers, zucchini, eggplant)
- 1/4 cup crumbled feta cheese
- 2 tablespoons chopped fresh herbs (e.g., parsley, basil)
- 2 tablespoons extra virgin olive oil
- 1 tablespoon lemon juice
- Salt and pepper to taste

Instructions:

- In a bowl, combine the cooked quinoa, roasted vegetables, crumbled feta cheese, and fresh herbs.

- In a separate small bowl, whisk together the olive oil, lemon juice, salt, and pepper to make the dressing.

- Drizzle the dressing over the quinoa salad and toss well to coat.

- Adjust the seasoning if needed.

- Pack the salad in a lunch container and refrigerate until ready to eat.

- Enjoy this nutrient-rich salad as a satisfying and flavorful lunch option.

2. Hummus and Veggie Wrap

Ingredients:

- Whole wheat tortilla or wrap

- 1/4 cup hummus

- Assorted fresh vegetables (e.g., cucumber, bell peppers, carrots, spinach)

- Sprouts or microgreens (optional)

- Salt and pepper to taste

Instructions:

- Spread the hummus evenly on the whole wheat tortilla or wrap.

- Layer the fresh vegetables and sprouts/microgreens on top of the hummus.

- Season with salt and pepper to taste.

- Tightly roll up the tortilla or wrap and slice it into smaller portions if desired.

- Pack the hummus and veggie wrap in a lunch container or wrap it in foil.

- It can be enjoyed as a fulfilling and nutritious lunch or snack on the go.

3. Energy-Boosting Trail Mix

Ingredients:

- 1 cup mixed nuts (e.g., almonds, walnuts, cashews)

- 1/2 cup dried fruits (e.g., raisins, cranberries, apricots)

- 1/4 cup dark chocolate chips or chunks

- 1/4 cup pumpkin seeds

- 1/4 cup unsweetened coconut flakes (optional)

Instructions:

- In a bowl, combine all the ingredients and mix well.

- Adjust the quantities according to your preferences.

- Portion the trail mix into small snack-sized containers or resealable bags.

- Carry these energy-packed snacks with you to enjoy throughout the day, whether at work, school, or during outdoor activities.

- Trail mix provides a combination of healthy fats, protein, and carbohydrates, making it a perfect on-the-go snack to keep you fueled and satisfied.

These power-packed lunch and snack ideas offer a balance of nutrients, flavors, and textures, providing sustained energy and promoting overall well-being.

Nourishing Dinners for Optimal Health

Here are three nourishing dinner ideas that promote optimal health:

1. Grilled Salmon with Roasted Vegetables

Ingredients:

- 4 salmon fillets
- 2 tablespoons olive oil
- 2 cloves garlic, minced
- 1 teaspoon lemon zest
- 1 teaspoon dried dill
- Salt and pepper to taste
- Assorted vegetables for roasting (e.g., broccoli, carrots, Brussels sprouts)

Instructions:

- Preheat your grill to medium-high heat.

- In a small bowl, combine the olive oil, minced garlic, lemon zest, dried dill, salt, and pepper to make a marinade.

- Place the salmon fillets in a shallow dish and pour the marinade over them, making sure to coat all sides.

- Let the salmon marinate for about 15-20 minutes.

- Meanwhile, preheat your oven to 425°F (220°C).

- Toss the assorted vegetables with olive oil, salt, and pepper in a baking dish.

- Roast the vegetables in the preheated oven for about 20-25 minutes, or until they are tender and slightly browned.

- While the vegetables are roasting, grill the salmon fillets for about 4-5 minutes per side, or until cooked through.

- Serve the grilled salmon alongside the roasted vegetables for a delicious and nutrient-rich dinner.

2. Quinoa Stir-Fry with Tofu and Vegetables

Ingredients:

- 1 cup cooked quinoa

- 1 block firm tofu, drained and cubed

- Assorted vegetables, sliced (e.g., bell peppers, broccoli, snap peas)

- 2 tablespoons low-sodium soy sauce

- 1 tablespoon sesame oil

- 2 cloves garlic, minced

- 1 teaspoon grated ginger

- 1 tablespoon sesame seeds (optional)

- Salt and pepper to taste

Instructions:

- In a large skillet or wok, heat the sesame oil over medium heat.

- Add the minced garlic and grated ginger to the skillet and sauté for about 1 minute until fragrant.

- Add the cubed tofu and cook until it starts to turn golden brown on all sides.

- Add the sliced vegetables to the skillet and stir-fry for about 3-4 minutes until they are crisp-tender.

- In a small bowl, whisk together the low-sodium soy sauce, salt, and pepper.

- Push the tofu and vegetables to one side of the skillet and add the cooked quinoa to the other side.

- Pour the soy sauce mixture over the quinoa and stir everything together to combine.

- Cook for an additional 1-2 minutes until everything is heated through.

- Sprinkle with sesame seeds for added crunch and flavor, if desired.

- Serve the quinoa stir-fry hot as a well-balanced and satisfying dinner option.

3. Baked Chicken Breast with Roasted Sweet Potatoes and Steamed Greens

Ingredients:

- 4 boneless, skinless chicken breasts

- 2 tablespoons olive oil

- 1 teaspoon garlic powder

- 1 teaspoon paprika

- Salt and pepper to taste

- 2 medium sweet potatoes, peeled and cubed

- Assorted greens (e.g., kale, spinach, Swiss chard)

Instructions:

- Preheat your oven to 425°F (220°C).

- Place the chicken breasts on a baking sheet lined with parchment paper.

- Drizzle the chicken breasts with olive oil and sprinkle with garlic powder, paprika, salt, and pepper. Rub the seasonings into the chicken to ensure even coating.

- In a separate bowl, toss the cubed sweet potatoes with olive oil, salt, and pepper.

- Spread the sweet potatoes in a single layer on another baking sheet lined with parchment paper.

- Place both the chicken breasts and the sweet potatoes in the preheated oven. Bake for about 20-25 minutes, or until the chicken is cooked through and the sweet potatoes are tender and lightly browned.

- While the chicken and sweet potatoes are baking, prepare the steamed greens. Fill a pot with a few inches of water and place a steamer basket inside.

- Bring the water to a boil. Add the greens to the steamer basket, cover the pot, and steam for about 3-5 minutes, or until the greens are wilted and tender.

- Once the chicken, sweet potatoes, and greens are cooked, remove them from the oven and stove top.

- Let the chicken rest for a few minutes before slicing it.

- Serve the baked chicken breasts with roasted sweet potatoes and steamed greens on the side.

- Season with additional salt and pepper if needed.

- Enjoy your nourishing dinner!

This meal provides lean protein from the chicken, complex carbohydrates from the sweet potatoes, and a dose of vitamins and minerals from the steamed greens. It's a well-rounded and nutritious option for a healthy dinner.

4. Grilled Chicken Breast with Quinoa and Steamed Broccoli

Ingredients:

- 4 boneless, skinless chicken breasts

- 2 tablespoons olive oil

- 1 teaspoon garlic powder

- 1 teaspoon paprika

- Salt and pepper to taste

- 1 cup cooked quinoa

- 2 cups broccoli florets

Instructions:

- Preheat your grill or stovetop grill pan over medium-high heat.

- Drizzle the chicken breasts with olive oil and season with garlic powder, paprika, salt, and pepper on both sides.

- Grill the chicken breasts for about 6-8 minutes per side, or until cooked through.

- While the chicken is grilling, prepare the quinoa according to the package instructions.

- Steam the broccoli florets until tender, about 5-7 minutes.

- Serve the grilled chicken with a side of cooked quinoa and steamed broccoli for a well-balanced meal.

5. Baked Salmon with Roasted Brussels Sprouts and Sweet Potatoes

Ingredients:

- 4 salmon fillets

- 2 tablespoons olive oil

- 2 cloves garlic, minced

- 1 teaspoon lemon zest

- Salt and pepper to taste

- 2 cups Brussels sprouts, halved

- 2 medium sweet potatoes, peeled and cubed

- 1 tablespoon balsamic vinegar

Instructions:

- Preheat your oven to 400°F (200°C).

- Place the salmon fillets on a baking sheet lined with parchment paper.

- In a small bowl, combine the olive oil, minced garlic, lemon zest, salt, and pepper. Brush the mixture onto the salmon fillets.

- In a separate bowl, toss the halved Brussels sprouts and cubed sweet potatoes with olive oil, salt, and pepper.

- Spread the Brussels sprouts and sweet potatoes on another baking sheet.

- Place both baking sheets in the preheated oven and bake for about 20-25 minutes, or until the salmon is cooked through and the vegetables are tender.

- Drizzle the roasted vegetables with balsamic vinegar before serving.

6. Lentil Curry with Brown Rice and Sautéed Spinach

Ingredients:

- 1 cup dried lentils, rinsed and drained

- 1 tablespoon olive oil

- 1 onion, diced

- 2 cloves garlic, minced

- 1 tablespoon curry powder

- 1 teaspoon ground cumin

- 1 teaspoon ground coriander

- 1 can (14 oz) diced tomatoes

- 1 cup vegetable broth

- Salt and pepper to taste

- 2 cups cooked brown rice

- 4 cups fresh spinach

Instructions:

- Cook the lentils according to the package instructions until tender.

- In a large skillet, heat the olive oil over medium heat.

- Add the diced onion and minced garlic to the skillet and sauté until the onion is translucent.

- Stir in the curry powder, cumin, and coriander, and cook for another minute.

- Add the diced tomatoes with their juice and vegetable broth to the skillet. Bring to a simmer.

- Stir in the cooked lentils and season with salt and pepper. Simmer for about 10-15 minutes to allow the flavors to meld together.

- In a separate skillet, sauté the spinach until wilted.

- Serve the lentil curry over brown rice, with a side of sautéed spinach.

These dinner ideas provide a balance of protein, healthy fats, fiber, and a variety of vitamins and minerals for optimal health. Enjoy!

Chapter 11

Putting It All Together: Creating Your Personalized Disease-Fighting Diet

"Creating Your Personalized Disease-Fighting Diet" focuses on creating a personalized eating routine that takes into account a person's particular health requirements and tries to bolster the body's defenses against diseases. This strategy aims to strengthen the immune system and advance general wellbeing by taking into account elements including medical history, genetic predispositions, lifestyle selections, and nutritional needs. A customized disease-fighting diet consists of nutrient-balanced meals, specific foods with disease-fighting qualities, and the avoidance of trigger foods. The customized plan is optimized for health outcomes with the help of a healthcare professional, like a registered dietitian, and encourages people to actively protect their health.

Assess Your Nutritional Needs

Assessing your nutritional needs is an important step in maintaining a healthy and balanced diet. It involves understanding your individual requirements for essential nutrients based on factors such as age, sex, activity level, and specific health conditions. By assessing your nutritional needs, you can make informed choices about the types and quantities of foods to consume to meet your body's requirements.

There are various methods to assess your nutritional needs. One common approach is to consult with a registered dietitian or nutritionist who can evaluate your overall health, lifestyle, and dietary habits. They can provide personalized recommendations based on your specific needs and goals.

Another method is to track your food intake using a food diary or mobile applications that provide nutritional information. This allows you to analyze your daily nutrient intake, identify any deficiencies or excesses, and make adjustments accordingly. Additionally, tools like online nutrient calculators can help estimate your recommended daily intake of calories, macronutrients (carbohydrates, proteins, and fats), vitamins, and minerals.

Regularly reassessing your nutritional needs is important as they may change over time due to factors such as aging, pregnancy, or changes in activity level or health conditions. It's important to note that while assessing your nutritional needs can provide valuable insights, it's always advisable to seek professional guidance for a comprehensive and accurate evaluation.

Design a Balanced and Science-Backed Eating Plan

Designing a balanced and science-backed eating plan involves considering various factors to ensure optimal nutrition and overall health. The foundation of a healthy eating plan should include a variety of nutrient-dense foods. Aim to incorporate a wide range of fruits, vegetables, whole grains, lean proteins, and healthy fats into your daily meals. These foods provide essential vitamins, minerals, fiber, and phytochemicals that support overall well-being. By including a diverse array of nutrient-dense foods, you can ensure that you're meeting your body's nutritional needs.

Another important aspect of a balanced eating plan is portion control. Paying attention to portion sizes can help you maintain a healthy energy balance and prevent overeating. Use visual cues, such as the plate method, which involves filling half your plate with vegetables, a quarter with lean protein, and a quarter with whole grains or starchy vegetables. This approach helps to ensure a well-rounded meal that includes a balance of macronutrients and adequate servings of different food groups.

In designing your eating plan, it's important to focus on whole, unprocessed foods. These foods are minimally processed and retain their natural nutrients. They are generally lower in added sugars, unhealthy fats, and sodium compared to heavily processed options. By prioritizing whole foods such as fruits, vegetables, whole grains, and lean proteins, you can maximize your intake of essential nutrients and minimize the consumption of additives and unhealthy ingredients.

Customization is key when it comes to designing an eating plan. Consider your individual needs, preferences, and any specific dietary requirements or restrictions you may have. Factors such as age, sex, activity level, and health conditions can influence your nutritional needs. Listen to your body's hunger and fullness cues, and make adjustments to your eating plan accordingly. It's also important to stay hydrated by drinking plenty of water throughout the day and limiting the consumption of sugary beverages.

While it's beneficial to educate yourself about nutrition and make informed choices, seeking professional guidance can be highly valuable. Consulting a registered dietitian or nutritionist can provide you with personalized recommendations tailored to your specific needs and goals. They can help assess your nutritional needs, address any health concerns, and provide science-backed advice to support your overall well-being. Working with a professional can help you navigate the vast amount of nutrition information available and ensure that your eating plan is based on sound principles and evidence. Remember, finding a sustainable and balanced approach to eating is key to long-term success and overall health.

Overcoming Challenges and Maintaining Long-Term Success

Maintaining long-term success with a healthy eating plan can sometimes be challenging, but with the right strategies, it is achievable.

Here are some tips for overcoming challenges and staying on track:

1. Set realistic goals

Start by setting achievable goals that are specific, measurable, attainable, relevant, and time-bound (SMART). Break down your larger goals into smaller, manageable steps. This approach helps you stay motivated and allows for a sense of accomplishment along the way.

2. Practice mindful eating

Mindful eating involves paying attention to your food choices, eating slowly, and savoring each bite. It helps you develop a better relationship with food and enhances your awareness of hunger and fullness cues. By practicing mindful eating, you can make conscious choices, enjoy your meals, and avoid overeating.

3. Plan and prepare your meal

Planning and preparing your meals in advance can help you make healthier choices and avoid impulse decisions. Set aside time each week to plan your meals, create a shopping list, and prep ingredients. Having nutritious meals and snacks readily available can prevent you from reaching for less healthy options when you're hungry or busy.

4. Seek support and accountability

Surround yourself with a support system of family, friends, or like-minded individuals who share your health goals. They can provide encouragement, share healthy recipes, and offer support when faced with challenges. Additionally, consider joining support groups or seeking professional guidance from a registered dietitian or nutritionist to help you stay accountable and provide guidance along your journey.

5. Practice self-compassion

Remember that healthy eating is not about perfection but rather progress. Be kind to yourself and practice self-compassion if you have a setback or make an unhealthy choice. Instead of dwelling on mistakes, focus on getting back on track with your next meal or snack. Celebrate your successes, no matter how small, and learn from any challenges you encounter.

6. Stay active

Regular physical activity complements a healthy eating plan and contributes to overall well-being. Find activities you enjoy and make them a part of your routine. Whether it's walking, cycling, dancing, or playing a sport, staying active helps maintain a healthy weight, boosts mood, and supports your overall health goals.

Remember, healthy eating is a lifelong journey, and it's normal to face challenges along the way. Stay committed, be adaptable, and celebrate your progress. With perseverance and a positive mindset, you can overcome obstacles and maintain long-term success in your healthy eating journey.

Conclusion

Empowering yourself with nutrition is crucial for achieving lifelong health and well-being. By taking control of your nutrition, you can make informed choices that support your overall health. One important step is to educate yourself about nutrition. Stay updated with reliable sources of information and learn about the impact of different nutrients on your body. This knowledge will enable you to navigate through conflicting advice and make informed decisions about the foods you consume.

A key aspect of empowering yourself with nutrition is focusing on whole, nutrient-dense foods. Incorporate plenty of fruits, vegetables, whole grains, lean proteins, and healthy fats into your diet. These foods provide essential nutrients, vitamins, minerals, and fiber that are vital for your health. Aim for a varied and colorful diet to ensure you're getting a wide range of nutrients from different food sources.

Practicing moderation and balance is another important strategy. Avoid extreme diets or strict restrictions that can lead to nutrient deficiencies or an unhealthy relationship with food. Instead, adopt a balanced approach to eating by including all food groups in appropriate portions. Allow yourself occasional treats or indulgences while prioritizing overall nutrient density and portion control. This way, you can enjoy a wide variety of foods while still maintaining a healthy and balanced diet.

Listening to your body and developing a mindful connection with your eating habits is crucial. Pay attention to your body's hunger and fullness cues, and eat when you're truly hungry and stop when you're satisfied. Be mindful of how different foods make you feel and adjust your choices accordingly. This awareness will help you make conscious decisions about what you eat and how it impacts your overall well-being.

Making gradual and sustainable changes is key to long-term success. Instead of attempting drastic dietary overhauls, focus on implementing small, achievable changes over time. Set realistic goals and build upon them as you develop healthier habits. By taking small steps, you can create lasting changes that are easier to maintain and integrate into your lifestyle.

If you have specific health concerns or dietary restrictions, seeking professional guidance from a registered dietitian or nutritionist can be beneficial. They can provide personalized guidance, help you navigate nutritional challenges, and create a tailored plan to support your unique needs. Professional advice can be particularly helpful when addressing specific health conditions, managing weight, or optimizing athletic performance.

Remember that nutrition is a lifelong journey, and it's never too late to start making positive changes. Empowering yourself with nutrition knowledge and adopting a balanced approach to eating will allow you to take charge of your health and well-being, supporting you in leading a fulfilling and healthy life.

The Journey towards Disease Prevention and Reversal

The journey towards disease prevention and reversal is an empowering and transformative process that puts you in control of your health. It starts with understanding that many chronic diseases are influenced by lifestyle factors, including diet and physical activity. By making positive changes to these aspects of your life, you can reduce your risk of developing certain diseases and even reverse existing conditions.

A key component of the journey is adopting a whole-food, plant-based diet. This approach focuses on consuming predominantly unprocessed plant foods such as fruits, vegetables, whole grains, legumes, nuts, and seeds. These foods are rich in fiber, antioxidants, vitamins, and minerals that support optimal health and provide protection against various diseases. By centering your meals on plants and minimizing or eliminating processed and animal-based foods, you can significantly enhance your overall well-being.

Regular physical activity is another vital aspect of the journey towards disease prevention and reversal. Engaging in regular exercise helps to maintain a healthy weight, improve cardiovascular health, strengthen muscles and bones, and enhance mental well-being. Find activities that you enjoy and make them a regular part of your routine. Whether it's brisk walking, cycling, swimming, or participating in group fitness classes, finding ways to stay active will have a profound impact on your health.

In addition to dietary and exercise changes, managing stress levels and getting sufficient sleep are essential for disease prevention and reversal. Chronic stress and inadequate sleep can have detrimental effects on your immune system, hormone balance, and overall health. Incorporating stress-reduction techniques such as meditation, deep breathing exercises, or engaging in activities that bring you joy and relaxation can help mitigate the negative effects of stress.

Prioritizing restful sleep and establishing healthy sleep habits will also support your body's natural healing and rejuvenation processes.

The journey towards disease prevention and reversal is not always easy, and it requires dedication, perseverance, and support. Surround yourself with a supportive network of family, friends, or even healthcare professionals who can offer guidance, encouragement, and accountability.

Celebrate your successes along the way, no matter how small, and be patient with yourself as you navigate through any challenges or setbacks. Remember that every positive step you take towards a healthier lifestyle is a step towards preventing and even reversing disease, allowing you to live a vibrant and fulfilling life.

Goodluck!!!

References

Boehm, K., Borrelli, F., Ernst, E., Habacher, G., Hung, S. K., Milazzo, S., ... & Schmidt, B. M. (2009). Green tea (Camellia sinensis) for the prevention of cancer. Cochrane Database of Systematic Reviews, (3).

Carr, A., & Maggini, S. (2017). Vitamin C and immune function. Nutrients, 9(11), 1211.

Fisberg, M., Machado, R., Koch, V., & Fisberg, R. M. (2018). Comparative analysis of the nutritional quality of yogurts consumed in Brazil: A useful tool for preventing cardiovascular diseases. Journal of Clinical Lipidology, 12(2), 549.

Fulgoni, V. L., Dreher, M., & Davenport, A. J. (2013). Avocado consumption is associated with better diet quality and nutrient intake, and lower metabolic syndrome risk in US adults: Results from the National Health and Nutrition Examination Survey (NHANES) 2001-2008. Nutrition Journal, 12(1), 1-9.

Gajendragadkar, P. R., Hubsch, A., & Mäki-Petäjä, K. M. (2014). Effects of oral lycopene supplementation on vascular function in patients with cardiovascular disease and healthy volunteers: A randomised controlled trial. PloS One, 9(6), e99070.

Gomes, A. C., et al. (2018). The role of gut microbiota modulation in the management of metabolic syndrome. Nutrition, 59, 20-35.

Grzanna, R., Lindmark, L., & Frondoza, C. G. (2005). Ginger—an herbal medicinal product with broad anti-inflammatory actions. Journal of Medicinal Food, 8(2), 125-132.

Haro, C., et al. (2016). Intestinal microbiota, obesity and metabolic syndrome. Molecular Nutrition & Food Research, 61(1), 1-13.

https://alchetron.com/Methanobrevibacter

https://commons.m.wikimedia.org/wiki/File:DIETA_MEDI TERRANEA_ITALIA.JPG Photo by G.steph.rocket:

https://en.m.wikipedia.org/wiki/Mediterranean_diet

https://seniorstoday.in/food/the-benefits-of-superfoods

https://upload.wikimedia.org/wikipedia/commons/1/12/Har vard_food_pyramid.png Walter C. Willett, M.D.

https://www.biocodex.com/en/about-us/biocodex-heritage/

https://www.britannica.com/science/nutrition/Lipids-fats-and-oils

https://www.cdc.gov/chronicdisease/resources/publications/
factsheets/nutrition.htm#

https://www.insularlife.com.ph/articles/the-benefits-of-
eating-healthy-food-00000157

https://www.medicaldaily.com/ancient-virus-crassphage-
lives-half-all-intestines-could-lead-obesity-diabetes-
drugs-294668

https://www.msdmanuals.com/home/disorders-of-
nutrition/overview-of-nutrition/overview-of-
nutrition#

https://www.ncbi.nlm.nih.gov/pmc/articles/PMC4290017/

https://www.news-medical.net/news/20220613/Gut-
microbiome-may-be-the-black-box-of-nutrition-
research.aspx

https://www.supplementsglobal.com/product/bifidobacteriu
m-bifidum/

https://www.taste.com.au/galleries/top-25-recipes-healthy-
gut/0ou63leo

Jurenka, J. S. (2008). Therapeutic applications of
pomegranate (Punica granatum L.): A review.
Alternative Medicine Review, 13(2), 128-144.

Khan, Z., Bhadouria, P., & Bisen, P. S. (2005). Nutritional
and therapeutic potential of spirulina. Current
Pharmaceutical Biotechnology, 6(5), 373-379.

Koushik, A., Hunter, D. J., Spiegelman, D., Beeson, W. L.,
van den Brandt, P. A., Buring, J. E., ... &
Giovannucci, E. L. (2007). Fruits, vegetables, and
colon cancer risk in a pooled analysis of 14 cohort

studies. Journal of the National Cancer Institute, 99(19), 1471-1483.

Latif, R. (2013). Chocolate/cocoa and human health: A review. Netherlands Journal of Medicine, 71(2), 63-68.

Paramsothy, S., et al. (2017). Multidonor intensive faecal microbiota transplantation for active ulcerative colitis: a randomised placebo-controlled trial. The Lancet, 389(10075), 1218-1228.

Rahman, K. (2007). Effects of garlic on platelet biochemistry and physiology. Molecular Nutrition & Food Research, 51(11), 1335-1344.

Ros, E. (2010). Health benefits of nut consumption. Nutrients, 2(7), 652-682.

Satija, A., Bhupathiraju, S. N., Rimm, E. B., Spiegelman, D., Chiuve, S. E., Borgi, L., ... & Hu, F. B. (2016). Plant-based dietary patterns and incidence of type 2 diabetes in US men and women: Results from three prospective cohort studies. PLOS Medicine, 13(6), e1002039.

Slyepchenko, A., et al. (2017). Gut emotions - mechanisms of action of probiotics as novel therapeutic targets for depression and anxiety disorders. CNS & Neurological Disorders-Drug Targets, 16(8), 919-933.

Sun, B., Ricardo-da-Silva, J. M., & Spranger, I. (2010). Critical factors of vegetables for health-promotion: Broccoli as a case study. Critical Reviews in Food Science and Nutrition, 50(9), 854-873.)

Swanson, D., Block, R., & Mousa, S. A. (2012). Omega-3 fatty acids EPA and DHA: Health benefits throughout life. Advances in Nutrition, 3(1), 1-7.

Vega-Gálvez, A., Miranda, M., Vergara, J., Uribe, E., Puente, L., & Martínez, E. A. (2010). Nutrition facts and functional potential of quinoa (Chenopodium quinoa Willd.), an ancient Andean grain: A review. Journal of the Science of Food and Agriculture, 90(15), 2541-2547.

Vuksan, V., Choleva, L., Jovanovski, E., Jenkins, A. L., Au-Yeung, F., Dias, A. G., ... & Sievenpiper, J. L. (2017). Comparison of flaxseed and chia seed consumption on inflammation and oxidative stress in overweight adults. Journal of the American College of Nutrition, 36(1), 9-15.)

Wasser, S. P. (2017). Medicinal mushrooms as a source of antitumor and immunomodulating polysaccharides. Applied Microbiology and Biotechnology, 101(3), 881-891.

Yokoyama, Y., Barnard, N. D., Levin, S. M., & Watanabe, M. (2017). Vegetarian diets and glycemic control in diabetes: A systematic review and meta-analysis. Cardiovascular Diagnosis and Therapy, 7(Suppl 1), S52-S62.